When an end-of-life conditi~~~ ~~~~ups, depression, confusion, and misunderstanding prevail among the patients, physicians, nurses, and families. The tragedy is that the spirit often dies before the patient. Insight into a solution to this spiritual failure is ably provided by Judy Flickinger, RN, in her book. Through her stories and lessons, the author demonstrates how the patient's treatment can be modified and the environment adjusted to restore the failing spirit. Flickinger shares her experience and knowledge in guiding the patient, family, and medical personnel to a positive outcome. This book is important reading for every one of us, including those in the medical field.

—J. Gerald Toole, MD

I've always thought that the people who work for hospice are at least part angel. Judy Flickinger is no exception. She's used her experiences with dying people, her insight, and her wisdom to provide sound and uplifting advice for people in the final phase of their lives. I highly recommend this book for both caregivers and for people who want to stay truly alive until the very end.

—Hal Urban, PhD, author, *Life's Greatest Lessons*

Judy Flickinger courageously confronts our final phase of life with wisdom and compassion.

—Larry Dossey, MD, author of eleven books, including *The Power of Premonitions* and *Healing Words*

When we truly accept our mortality, we learn about life. The best hospices have graduations and dropouts because when people get ready to die, they truly can begin to learn to live. The lessons to be learned from this book will help you to live, fully alive. Your life can be enhanced by its wisdom and the author's insight into the human spirit.

—Bernie Siegel, MD, author of eleven books, including *365 Prescriptions for the Soul,* and *Faith, Hope, & Healing*

Spirit Matters

Spirit Matters

How to Remain *Fully Alive*
with a Life-Limiting Illness

Judy Flickinger

TATE PUBLISHING *& Enterprises*

Published by Tate Publishing & Enterprises, LLC
127 E. Trade Center Terrace | Mustang, Oklahoma 73064 USA
1.888.361.9473 | www.tatepublishing.com

Tate Publishing is committed to excellence in the publishing industry. The company reflects the philosophy established by the founders, based on Psalm 68:11,
"The Lord gave the word and great was the company of those who published it."

Book design copyright © 2009 by Tate Publishing, LLC. All rights reserved.
Cover design by Amber Gulilat
Interior design by Lindsay B. Behrens

Published in the United States of America

ISBN: 978-1-61566-784-0
1. Medical / Terminal Care   2. Body, Mind & Spirit / Healing / General
09.12.16

Dedication

To the many families for whom I had the privilege of providing end-of- life care during my hospice career. Thank you for inviting me into your lives when you were so vulnerable. Our time together changed my life forever and filled me with the knowledge and inspiration to write this book.

Acknowledgments

While I have many persons to thank, none deserves my gratitude as much as my husband. Through his countless hours of editing, while he might have changed my words, he never changed my message. Roger, I hope you know how much that meant to me. You are my soul mate and the love of my life. I know that this book would not have been possible without you.

My hospice career began with my mentors, Lila Van Cuyk and Pat Stropko-O'Leary. Thank you both for teaching me the true mission of hospice and being responsible for starting me on the right path.

When I decided to write this book, Billie Robinson took my notes and typed for hours on end, compiling them all into a single file. Thank you, Billie, for your hard work and for your friendship over all these years.

Thanks to Mary Jane Skala, who reviewed the original draft and graciously shared her expertise and editorial suggestions. Roger took over from there, and after innumerable hours of editing and reorganizing, we finally produced what we thought was a finished manuscript. A final review by Dr. Joan West provided some needed polish and was greatly appreciated.

Thanks also to Phyllis Fliess for the support and motivation she provided during my seemingly endless search for a publisher.

I would be remiss if I didn't say a special thank you to Jane Gentry, the best former daughter-in-law and friend a person could ask for. There were many times when she encouraged me and cheered me on when the task seemed overwhelming.

And finally, thank you to the many friends, family members, and of course, my children for their love and encouragement.

Table of Contents

Foreword

Hospice and end-of-life care have become part of my personal mission since the death of my father. Unfortunately, in our modern medical system, misinformation and misunderstanding about end-of-life issues are often the rule rather than the exception. Although treatment for disease has advanced dramatically in the last half century, acceptance of death as a part of life has not. While we often over treat dying patients, we underestimate their need for honesty about their decline.

This book deeply reflects what I do every day in my practice as a hospice medical director. When I speak with patients and their loved ones, I am sincere, compassionate, and honest. People are often shocked because their own physician had not told them the seriousness of their condition. Although terminal, most people can hear the truth more easily than promises of aggressive treatments that are no longer viable but are often debilitating. They are often relieved when I tell them that the time has come to move them from aggressive curative care to aggressive comfort care.

Spirit Matters is the first book I've seen that focuses on the overlooked importance of keeping the spirit, the "person" inside the dying body, healthy during the course of a life-limiting illness. Although written primarily for the layperson, health care professionals will also gain a new perspective on what really matters at the end of life—the often missed but ultimately most important ingredient in end-of-life care is a person's spirit.

Judy Flickinger brings her own unique perspective to the subject from her twelve years as a hospice nurse and now as a hospice volunteer. Her writing style and personal stories bring about tears as well as laughter and inspiration. This book can help change the way we as Americans view this natural part of life that we often find so difficult to face. It is only when we embrace all parts of life that we allow ourselves to live every minute fully and joyfully.

—Segismundo Pares, MD
Senior Medical Director, Hospice of Marion County
Medical Director, Center for Comprehensive
Palliative Care, 2008 recipient of Florida Hospital
Association "Hospital Hero" award for palliative care

Introduction

Horace Mann once said, "We should be ashamed to die without some contribution to humanity."

This book, hopefully, will be my contribution. It is intended to teach you some important truths that I believe you will want to know when your time comes to deal with a life-limiting illness, be it your own or that of a loved one.

Spirit Matters is about helping people live full and productive lives while they are dying. It focuses on the importance of keeping the spirit—the person inside the dying body—alive and well during the course of a terminal illness. It brings hope and assurance that the end of life does not have to be a physically painful, frightening, and isolated experience. Most importantly, it will educate and empower the dying and their loved ones to take control of crucial decisions that are typically left to medical and bureaucratic systems that have little understanding of the real needs of the dying person.

Spirit Matters offers a seldom-considered but all-important perspective on what really matters at the end of life; in far too many cases a person's spirit is destroyed long before the body dies.

Life is terminal! We will all die, but our youth-oriented society finds this hard to accept and lives mostly in denial of this basic fact of life. Even when confronted with the inescapable reality of a terminal illness, we often try to pretend that it is not happening by adopting a variety of defenses. At first, we may downplay or even ignore the condition. Or we may take a "fight on, regardless" attitude in an unrealistic grasp at a miracle medical straw. In an attempt to shield our fragile emotions and egos from the inevitable truth, we may avoid talking honestly about the impending death. Not just the dying and their loved ones but also physicians, nurses, social workers, and even some clergy succumb to these all-too-human but misguided responses. As a result, we fail to learn and understand what is truly important in the life of the dying person.

If we are not knowledgeable and prepared to communicate our desires before the fact, it becomes very difficult to be in control of our dying. When the dying or those around them are reluctant or afraid to talk about or deal realistically with a life-limiting illness before it is too late, a priceless opportunity is wasted, and the dying may lose much, if not all, of their power to influence how they spend their final time. As they approach the end, the dying have less and less energy to make their wants and needs known and to deal with the difficult issues that inevitably arise. By default, they are forced to leave crucial decisions to those they hope know best and have their best interests at heart.

Unfortunately, if the issues weren't discussed earlier, those people (usually physicians or family members), even though well meaning, often have no real understanding of what the dying need or want, and it becomes their own, not the dying person's, interests that are promoted. In today's society, where some people insist that delaying death is more important than quality of life and reduction of suffering, the spirit is at severe risk for prolonged distress if the wrong people are making the decisions.

Dying people are often pressured into accepting aggressive treatments that are not only physically and spiritually debilitating but also ultimately futile. Why do we do this? Why do we allow it to happen? Why is good terminal care not common practice even though it is readily available? Why do we persist in denying terminally ill patients the end-of-life care that can provide the physical and emotional comfort that allows the spirit to be healed (or prevents it from being destroyed in the first place)? Unfortunately, there are many reasons. Fear, denial, pride, money, ignorance, egotistical medical attitudes, and a litigation-prone society are all responsible to one degree or another.

With the availability of modern medical technology, we can forestall death. We can demand one more procedure or one more treatment that might somehow bring about a miraculous cure. For better or worse, many in the medical profession readily support us in this position. Physicians often find it difficult to admit that there is nothing more medically that they can do. Their focus is on cure, and most of them have had little training in end-of-life care. Also, although you won't find many who will admit to it as a cause, life-prolonging treatments and procedures, although often ultimately futile, can make a lot of money for hospitals, physicians, and nursing homes.

If not properly treated, the physical symptoms, such as pain and nausea, and the emotional distress caused by a terminal disease or aggressive attempts to cure it can be overwhelming. Recovery and healing of one's spirit are not possible under such conditions, yet by the time we finally admit that the body cannot be cured, there is often very little left of the person inside. Even worse, precious time is wasted and lost forever, scarce time that could have been better spent nurturing and enriching the dying person's spirit so that the remaining life might have some quality and meaning for both the patient and the loved ones. When proper care and treatment are provided to alleviate the physical and emotional suffering, the spirit will have a chance to remain fully alive.

Ignorance bears a large responsibility for poor end-of-life care. Time and again I have seen unnecessary despair and suffering simply because people didn't know that it didn't have to be that way. Far more than they dreamed possible can be done when faced with a terminal illness. You don't have to just give up and die. You don't have to accept the disabling pain and nausea and diarrhea and constipation and the countless other afflictions that might beset you. You can be taught how to manage the debilitating fatigue, loss of appetite, and the many other symptoms that can occur with a life-limiting illness. Much can be accomplished, and many people have been able to maintain productive lives right up until the end.

It is not necessary to let your spirit die before your body does. However, you can't expect this to happen by good luck or chance. Being unprepared, uninformed, and uneducated about death and dying are some of the most unfortunate circumstances that can happen when faced with a life-limiting illness. We normally plan for everything: college, careers, weddings, babies, birthday parties, retirement—everything but how we are going to deal with our deaths.

As I noted earlier, we don't want to talk about "it." I also hid from "it" until I became a hospice nurse and saw firsthand the devastation caused by ignorance and avoidance, and just the opposite, how wonderful and fulfilling an end-of-life experience can be for all those involved when time, proper care, and support are provided.

What can be done to change our attitudes and give us the chance for a positive end-of-life experience? The lessons and stories contained in the following chapters will provide the insight needed to make this happen.

I am not a writer by profession. I am a nurse with forty years of professional experience, the last twelve years as a hospice nurse caring for people with life-limiting illnesses. Hospice nurses spend much of their time teaching loved ones how to care for their patients and teaching those patients how to let go of life. During my career in hospice, my patients and their loved ones also taught me many important truths about dying—far more than I ever taught them. This book is about what we taught each other and how I learned that there is a difference between the act of dying and the art of dying.

Although hospice is not the primary theme of *Spirit Matters*, since it plays such an integral role in developing my message, it will be helpful if you have a basic understanding of what hospice is all about. Hospice is a program for taking care of people who have terminal illnesses. It should not be looked at as a place where people go to die but rather as a philosophy of care that emphasizes living your life to the fullest in the time that remains. It does not necessarily mean that you are going to die soon; I have had patients who continued to work, travel, go out with friends, and do any number of things that are a part of normal living.

Entering a hospice program does mean, however, that your illness cannot be cured and that the time you have left is limited. A person ready for hospice might say, "If there is no cure for my disease and I do not want to be placed on life support should I become incapacitated or stop breathing, then let me be cared for in my own home or in a homelike setting where my treatment will be for comfort care until my death."

The criteria for hospice care are not complicated or difficult to meet. They are:

1. A diagnosis of a life-limiting illness with an expected life span of six months or less (if the disease takes its normal course)

2. A physician's order for hospice care

3. The patient's awareness of the prognosis (if he or she is cognizant) and the desire not to be resuscitated or placed on life support, which may be stated in a living will

4. The patient's acknowledgment that treatment with intent to cure will be discontinued and replaced with treatment to provide comfort

Hospice programs are carried out by teams of dedicated medical and social professionals and volunteers and can be found almost anywhere in the country in the local phone book or on the Internet. While some have in-patient facilities, and many nursing homes also offer in-house hospice, most of the end-of-life care provided by hospice is in the patient's home. Regardless of where it takes place, hospice is an entitlement for Medicare and state Medicaid terminally ill patients. Also, most private insurance plans have a hospice benefit. Hospice patients are not charged for this service.

Many of my hospice families have told me, "Judy, please tell our story so that others can learn what we wish we had known." This book is my promise to do just that. Its message is presented through lessons illustrated by the personal stories of dying people I have known and cared for. In each chapter or lesson, I address a particular issue related to what is truly important at the end of life. The themes overlap in places, as do the messages in the stories. Some of the stories could easily fit into a different lesson from where I placed them; the end-of-life experience has many common aspects.

Most of the stories relate to the experience of one family or person. A few are composites of similar circumstances. In consideration of personal and family privacy, some of the names and places have been changed. Regardless, they are all true accounts of the triumph of the human spirit. My hope is that you, the reader, will find them helpful in keeping you fully alive if you are ever coping with a terminal illness.

When you study these lessons and read the stories, laugh, cry, and be inspired as I was (and still am) by the courage and dedication of the people who lived them.

LESSON 1

My Spirit Is Who I Am

We are spirits. That bodies should be lent to us while they afford us pleasure, assist us in acquiring knowledge or in doing good to our fellow-creatures, is a kind of benevolent act of God. When they become unfit for these purposes and afford us pain instead of pleasure, instead of an aid become an encumbrance and answer none of these intentions for which they were given, it is equally kind and benevolent that a way is provided by which we get rid of them. Death is that way.

Benjamin Franklin
Letter after the death of his brother, 1756

Webster's Dictionary defines *spirit* as:

1. A vital principle held to give life to physical organism

2. Soul

3. The activating essential principle influencing a person

I think there is an easier definition. My spirit is who I am as a person. It is not who I am as a body or my physical appearance, but who I am inside. It is what gives life to my physical body. Every one of us has a spirit. If our spirits are wounded, we find it difficult or impossible to be ourselves and to live our lives. Without our spirits, we are just lifeless, empty shells. Life is not just a beating heart or a warm body; there must also be a living spirit to complete us as human beings.

It is an undisputed fact that 100 percent of us will die. The issue as I see it, however, is not that we are going to die, but how we will live as we approach our deaths. Statistics show that 90 percent of adults will die of a chronic, lingering illness. Contrary to what we may hope for as the best way out, most of us will not be afforded a quick and easy death but will take weeks, months, or even more time to pass through the terminal stage of dying. This revelation should give us concern about the state of our spirits during this period because if our spirits are not alive and well, our remaining time becomes an enemy when it could have been a friend.

As the current medical system takes its usual approach to a life-limiting illness, it often ignores a patient's spirit as it focuses on attempts to cure the disease. The unfortunate result is that by the time we finally admit that healing the body is no longer possible, there is often very little left of the person inside; the spirit is destroyed long before the disease kills the body.

How I Know about the Spirit

At one time my spirit was nearly destroyed. I learned a great deal from that experience. It helped me to understand the importance of the human spirit in making us whole persons. This episode in my life occurred long before I became a hospice nurse. I believe, however, that it guided me into hospice nursing. It gave me the sensitivity and empathy to understand the remarkable differences that healthy spirits can make, not only in the lives of terminally ill persons, but also in the lives of their loved ones.

My ordeal made me aware of the devastation and depth of loss that occurs when a spirit is destroyed, whether a person is dying of a physical disease or dying inside, experiencing an emotional death as I did. Yes, I realize that there is ultimately a vast difference between struggling with a life-limiting illness and my suffering from a severe depression, but I know that in many ways, the effect on the spirit is the same.

I know firsthand how damaging a destroyed spirit can be. I know the emptiness one feels. When I lost my spirit, I became nothing but a hollow shell. I was an empty body with no quality to my life or any purpose for living. I felt as if I had died inside.

I know the pain of not wanting to live. I know the pain it caused the people who loved and cared about me. The pain of my wounded spirit was the worst pain I ever experienced.

I know the anxiety and fear that can overwhelm you when you feel your spirit—the very essence of your being—slipping away and you do not have the strength or the will to do anything about it.

I know the sadness, confusion, doubt, and frustration that fill every waking hour. I have endured the sense of being trapped, the inability to make decisions, and the loss of control over one's life that happens when your spirit is dying.

Because of my own experience, when I began my hospice work, I could recognize an injured spirit when I saw one. Often, it was not what patients said but how they presented themselves. I saw in them some of the same signs and symptoms that I once saw in myself. In the depth of my illness, I remember looking into a mirror and not recognizing the person I saw looking back at me. She was almost not there and was surely not the passionate, alive woman that used to be me. I recognized that same look when I saw it on my hospice patients' faces. They were worn down and worn out. I could hear the same sadness in their voices that used to be in mine. Helping them recapture their spirits and seeing them return to their former selves was a wonderful sight, just as it was for me to see myself return to who I was before I began losing my spirit.

Protecting Your Spirit

I have described what it is like to lose one's spirit in order to help you understand, as I do now, the importance of protecting that spirit. If I had protected my spirit from the destructive forces that were causing my depression, I would have avoided much needless suffering. I should have been the guardian of my spirit and could have been if I had known then what I know now.

From my hospice experience, I learned that you, the patient, must be the guardian of your own spirit. Even when you have been diagnosed with a terminal illness, others, even your loved ones, may still be mostly concerned with your physical condition. They may not appreciate how crucial a strong spirit is to your well-being and to your ability to confront your disease.

In the life of a seriously ill person, the focus of care is on the body and making it well. Much energy is devoted to this purpose, and the spirit can get lost in the process. What we fail to realize is that without healthy spirits, we really have nothing with which to fight the diseases that are assaulting our bodies. Your energy may already be low from the treatments and the concerns and symptoms associated with your illness. And the more ill you become, the less energy you may have to protect your spirit.

Don't be fooled! If something is affecting your body, your spirit will feel it as well and will react accordingly. Fortunately, the human spirit is not quickly or easily depleted, but it is possible for it to be chipped away one small piece at a time. In the beginning of your illness, you may not even be aware that your spirit is being affected because all of your attention and energy are centered on your illness and what to do about it. But as the disease progresses, if unrelieved pain and similarly distressing conditions take hold, your spirit can be overwhelmed before you realize what has happened. You need to be prepared to protect your spirit before that happens. It takes much less effort to maintain a healthy spirit than it does to recover a damaged one, and the longer you let it go, the harder it is to get it back. You may not have much control over the progression of your disease, but with a healthy spirit, you can have greater control over your life.

It is not easy to defend your spirit, but you can be prepared to fight for it. The information in this book will give you both hope and help for the task, and once you are knowledgeable and determined to protect your spirit, nothing can take it away from you. You must be the one who decides how far you are willing to let the ravages of your illness and treatments erode your spirit.

Set a limit and then do not allow anyone or anything to push you beyond it unless it is *your* decision alone to change it. You must also make sure that your loved ones are aware of your wants and needs and the limits you have set and that they will honor your wishes and speak up for you if you are unable to do so.

Throughout this book, the stories of the patients I have cared for will illustrate that it is never too late to mend a broken spirit—and never too early to be concerned about its welfare. It is my hope that as you read on, you will come to fully understand and appreciate the importance of this truth.

Mary Jane

I had been doing my usual rounds at the hospital the day I met Cheryl and Mary Jane. At the time, I didn't think what I did was anything of great significance; it was just a normal part of the way I did hospice. However, when I received Cheryl's letter after the death of her mother, I knew that something special had happened.

While walking down the hallway in our medical unit, I could see that the lady outside of room 200 was staring at me. I remember her being a tall, lovely, well-dressed woman about my age.

She approached me and said, "Excuse me, are you the hospice lady?" I replied that yes, I was from hospice. She said, "My name is Cheryl. I need someone to listen to me. I can't stand to see what is happening to my mother." She asked me if I would take a minute to speak with her.

I followed her into the room, where I saw Cheryl's mother, Mary Jane, for the first time.

Mary Jane was frail looking, gray haired, and had a tiny, wrinkled face. Both of her arms were tied to the side rails of her bed, and I saw the terror in her eyes as she looked up at me. It reminded me of the terror one sees in the eyes of a trapped animal. I gently took her hand in mine and told her my name. I said that Cheryl had asked me to meet with them to try to make things better for her. I told her I would be back to see her in a few minutes. With that, Cheryl and I walked down to the end of the hallway to an empty room. We sat down, and I listened quietly while Cheryl spoke.

Cheryl began by telling me why her mother was in the hospital. Mary Jane had been in a nursing home for the previous four years with a deteriorating heart condition. She was eighty-seven years old and had been brought to the hospital four days before with pneumonia. She was doing poorly and wasn't able to speak for herself. The only way the nurses could keep her from pulling her intravenous and feeding tubes out was to tie her arms to the side rails of her bed. Cheryl said that her mother was miserable being tied down. The doctor had told her that her mother needed this "care" if she was ever going to get better, and even with this treatment, her chance of recovery was poor.

Cheryl said, "My mother is dying. I know that. I just can't stand to watch what is happening to her. Her lungs are full of fluid, yet they keep pouring stuff into the feeding tube and giving her intravenous fluids. She keeps looking at me as if to tell me to do something. I don't want my mother to die with her arms tied to the bed. She is being tortured, and I don't know how to stop it. Can you please help me?"

As I listened, I thought sadly about how often this happened. What gave the medical profession the right to destroy the spirit of this dying, elderly little lady?

Just then, Molly, a social worker with whom I often worked, came into the room. She and I frequently agreed that this type of so-called care caused more grief than good. We also agreed that it was a huge waste of our Medicare and Medicaid dollars. Molly sat down with us, and we proceeded to explain to Cheryl that she was right. Her mother's condition was getting worse, and no, she didn't need to die like this. Within one hour we had a physician's order to change her mother's care from aggressive to "hospice in the hospital." The tubes were removed, and the other unsuccessful treatments were stopped.

Cheryl and I sat by Mary Jane's bedside and untied her arms. She raised them slowly and just looked at her hands. Cheryl gasped and took her mother's hand in hers. With tears in her eyes she said, "Mom, that's better, isn't it?"

Her mother smiled for the first time in four days as she responded to this *new* treatment. Seeing Mary Jane's "recovery" was a wonderful experience, proving that it is never too late to heal a broken spirit. All hospice had done was give Mary Jane comfort care and support Cheryl in the process.

Even though I spent only a short amount of time with Cheryl and her mother that day, I received this note from Cheryl one week later.

> Dear Judy,
>
> Thank you for your support and quick action as my mother was passing on last week. My only regret is that I did not realize sooner that hospice existed and could make the end of life a peaceful and pain-free time.
>
> I will forever be grateful that you helped get the tubes out so she could pass on in peace.
>
> Sincerely,
>
> Cheryl (Daughter of Mary Jane)

LESSON 2

Spirit Matters

> He was moribund and screaming—I had no
> morphine. I finally instinctively sat down on the
> bed and took him in my arms, and the screaming
> stopped. He died peacefully in my arms a few
> hours later. It was not the pleurisy that caused
> the screaming, but the loneliness.
>
> Archie Cochran

When there is no cure for a terminal disease, love and
care will nurture the human spirit. At this stage, we
need to reduce our emphasis on physical survival and
place our emphasis on spiritual survival. Keeping the
spirit alive and well allows us to come to the end of
life ready and hopefully willing to let go and move on
to death.

When we come to the end of life, accepting the fact
that some of our former hopes and dreams will never
be realized allows us to let go. When we are dying, if

we accept the reality of what is happening, we can deal with things as they are, not as we wish they could be. We can then move on to death with our spirits intact, not broken and left in pieces. When cure is not possible, the ego's powerful craving for physical immortality *must* be muted so that the spirit can live. In so doing, it is possible to find peace while we are dying.

When we can no longer treat the disease that a person has, we should always look for other ways to help. This is when spirit matters the most. Spiritual healing is not the same as physical healing even though when something affects the body (for good or bad), it invariably affects the spirit. The well-being of the human spirit has nothing to do with winning the battle against dying because ultimately, you aren't going to win. Spiritual healing is more about how the battle is fought.

When we connect with the sick and dying and share their experience, we can increase the wellness of their spirits. What else can be more important and valuable if the body cannot be cured? Whatever your last wishes are, as long as they are not illegal or immoral, you deserve, at the least, to have someone make an attempt to honor them.

I have knocked on a patient's neighbor's door at night looking for the beer that he is sure they will have for him. We have arranged (with much difficulty) to bring a young adult son from prison—in shackles and with a guard—to say goodbye and to express his remorse to his dying father.

Just when we think we know what another's dying wish will be, we often find that we really don't know.

Golda

Golda was bald from her chemotherapy. This had the unfortunate effect of exposing her large, protruding ears. Even though she weighed about seventy-five pounds and looked like an ad for famine relief, her smile warmed my heart.

She was often more interested in how my day was going than in her own illness. This was in sharp contrast to her husband, who couldn't wait for my arrival so that I could check *his* blood pressure and listen to *his* health issues. He was slightly overweight, but from what I could tell, he was able to get around and do whatever he wanted. Their large old frame house, which had been allowed to run down, reflected his attitude and lack of interest in caring for his wife.

They had a small, loving old dog named Mattie that was Golda's constant companion. Her husband didn't like the dog much and did little to care for it. It was winter, and instead of going out, the dog did her business behind the couch in the living room. Golda's husband apparently didn't think this was a problem since he never let the dog out or cleaned up after her.

The first time this happened, I asked her husband why he hadn't cleaned up the mess. He told me that he wanted to get rid of the dog, and if Golda didn't like it, she could clean up after her own dog. By this time, Golda was having problems taking care of her own bathroom needs and had neither the energy nor the stamina to let Mattie outside or to pick up after her. Thus began my first chore upon my visits to Golda's house. I would follow the smell coming from behind the couch and pick up after Mattie.

Golda spent her days and nights in her living room on a small, old, tattered loveseat that had become her ever-diminishing world. I offered more than once to help her to her bed or to order a hospital bed that could make her more comfortable, but she insisted on staying where she was. As we are dying, we lose control of so much of ourselves. This was her way of maintaining some control of her life. When I visited with her in her home, I most often sat on the floor beside her, holding her hand as we talked about her life and her dying.

Despite her circumstances, with Mattie's help, Golda's spirit was holding up reasonably well. Still, I could tell that something was missing but couldn't quite put my finger on it. Thinking back, I remember that often during those visits I would see her looking pensively at my hair. She had shown me pictures of herself before the chemotherapy. Before her illness, she had beautiful, long red hair that covered up her (as she considered them) unsightly ears.

The day before she died, I asked her, as I always did before leaving a patient's home, if there was anything else that I could do for her before I left that day. She glanced again at my hair and asked, "Judy, may I touch your hair?"

Then I understood, and it was all I could do to say yes without crying. This dear woman was grieving the loss of her hair and suffering from what it meant to her to be seen with her large ears and no hair to cover them. I told her to touch my hair any time she wanted. We laughed together as I took off my coat and resumed my place on the floor beside her. As we sat there and talked about the sadness of losing her hair and her life, I watched the tears flow down her cheeks as she caressed my hair.

Yes, spirit does matter, but it is often difficult to realize and understand what matters to the spirit. Being physically touched usually has a beneficial effect on a patient's spirit, but in this case it worked the other way around. Being able to touch my hair and having someone know and care about her loss provided the final ingredients for healing her spirit. Golda died the next day, and as the hospice team believed would happen, she died on that same old loveseat that represented her last bit of control.

Mary

This story begins with a hospice admission. The family consisted of Scott, a young man aged twenty, Jo-ann, his sister, age twenty-two, and their mother, Mary, a forty-five-year-old woman dying of cancer. The home where she would spend her final time was a small, red-brick house in a suburb outside of Cleveland, Ohio. The woman was about my age, and her children were about the ages of my sons.

I reflect on this because whenever I do hospice in a home with a background similar to my own, it makes me realize just how universal the human experience can be. Very often I find this to be a difficult situation for me. It stares me right in the face and says, *This could be you!*

My two sons and my daughter experienced a great deal of pain in their past, just as Scott and Jo-ann did. Each family had a bitter divorce as its legacy. I saw the pain in Scott's and Jo-ann's eyes just as I continued to see it in my own children. It reflected sadness for what they had lived through and how their childhoods had been scarred.

Both Mary and I had been abused by our husbands, and every family member had witnessed it. As mothers, both of us felt guilt for the pain to which our children had been subjected. When I first met Mary, she was dead inside. At one stage in my life I was also dead inside and could understand her emptiness at a deep level.

Mary was nearing the end of her battle with cancer. She was so tiny, a bare wisp of what I saw in the pictures in her home from years gone by. Those pictures also revealed a warm smile that no longer existed. She still had pretty brown eyes and short blond hair that was slowly growing back after her chemotherapy treatments. Actually, her hair was quite pretty; the rest of her was just so very frail and sad.

Scott and Jo-ann were both bright and good-looking young adults. Neither had attended college, but both had responsible jobs in the community. Jo-ann worked at a nearby mall in a major department store. She was an attractive girl with long blond hair and a beautiful smile—the image of her mother in younger days. She had a boyfriend named Jesse. He was supportive, but Jo-ann was concerned that he might get tired of her situation; she wasn't able to see him as often as he wanted. I let her know that hospice would provide a volunteer to stay with her mom so that she and Jesse could go out a couple of times a week. Hopefully this would help balance their lives and provide some normalcy in these abnormal circumstances.

Scott installed carpeting for a local flooring company. He was a tall, thin young man with strong features and big brown eyes. He didn't have a girlfriend, but he was involved in sports. A volunteer could stay with Mary to give Scott some recreation time as well. Fortunately, both Scott's and Jo-ann's employers were being cooperative regarding their mother's care and the amount of work they missed. They took turns taking time off, as someone had to be in the home at all times with Mary.

Their story touched my heart. Dad had divorced Mom when she was diagnosed with breast cancer three years before. With Dad gone, the three of them fought the good fight together. Now that the disease had won the physical battle, the kids would stay with Mom and be her caregivers.

The fear in the home was so intense I could feel it. There were no other family members in the area they could call on for help. These young adults, with support from hospice, were totally responsible for their mother's care.

"I'm so afraid I will hurt her. I don't think I can give my mom a bath and change her Depends." On and on they went with their concerns and fears.

The fear that arises when going into the uncharted territory of death and dying can be contagious and overwhelming. It was my job to help Scott and Jo-ann work through some of those fears. We had a long talk when we met that first day. I told them hospice would teach them how to take care of their mother and that we would support them along the way. We all bonded quickly, and I assured them that they would not have to do this difficult task alone.

After admitting Mary to our hospice program, I presented her case at our weekly team meeting. I reported that I believed Mary's main problem was depression. I suggested to our medical director (a physician) that I should call Mary's physician and discuss this with him. Our medical director looked at me and exclaimed, "Why would you want to do that? Of course she's depressed. She's dying. Wouldn't you be depressed if you were dying? Why would you want to take that away from her?"

I bit my tongue as I answered, "It's our responsibility to help our patients find comfort. Emotional pain can be just as debilitating as physical pain. Terminally ill patients need their pain managed and relieved whether it is physical or emotional."

It was clear that he was angry with me as he dismissed it as a nonissue.

Understanding as I did the emotional pain of a depressed spirit, I knew I had to do something. After the meeting, I telephoned Mary's physician and explained my findings. Agreeing with me, he ordered an antidepressant for Mary. I nearly lost my job over this, but it was worth it as I watched Mary's spirit respond to the medication.

When I first began visits to her home, Mary was still able to get out of bed by herself. That changed as her condition declined. Scott and Jo-ann soon became totally responsible for all aspects of their mother's care. While they were trying to figure out how to be grown-ups, they also had to figure out how to cope with the care and inevitable death of their mother. They were willing and able students, just scared. Together we worked on those fears each time I visited their home.

As the hospice workers taught them and affirmed their care-giving abilities, they developed the confidence to do it themselves. Sometimes we had to show them different aspects of Mary's care over and over again, but once they were sure of their ability, they did a wonderful job.

As Mary became more ill, hospice began to add more support for her care. A nurse's aide began coming to the home daily to bathe Mary. Mary bonded with her volunteer, which made it emotionally easier for her children to leave her and go out occasionally with friends. Our social worker began meeting with the family to help sort out some of their personal issues and financial concerns. Now that hospice was supplying all of Mary's medications, the family's financial burdens were reduced.

Mary's symptoms due to her cancer were not that difficult to manage. The three of them—Mary, Scott, and Jo-ann—along with her physician, trusted my suggestions and saw good results. It seemed to me that most of my visits were spent in emotional comfort care. I listened—they talked.

As Mary became confined to her bed, I understood that most of her pain was emotional. She had already lost her husband, and now, in losing her life, she would also lose her children. Mary lay on her side while we talked, and I rubbed her back. I could feel her body relaxing as she told me her story. She talked often about her sadness and the dreams she had for her children. She was sad that she would not see her children marry and have children of their own. She talked about her former husband and how he had been emotionally abusive all of their marriage. The final abuse occurred when she found him with another woman after she had been diagnosed with cancer. She said that was "the straw that broke the camel's back."

I always connected with my hospice patients at some level, but my emotional and spiritual bond with this family was different. I believe what happened next was because of that bond. In my twelve years of hospice nursing, I had never gone to a home without calling first—except this once.

The day that Mary died, I was driving to another home, but something moved me to go to her home first. The feeling was so intense that I can remember thinking, *I need to get there right now.* It was clear that this was the right thing to do. As I pulled into her driveway and started toward the door, Scott and

Jo-ann came running out, crying. "Judy, how did you know? *Mom just died!*"

There was no doubt in my mind that our spirits were connected at some deeper level. I don't believe this could have happened if Mary's spirit hadn't recovered and strengthened during our time together. From one mother to another, I just knew that she wanted me to be there for her children. Did it happen because all of their spirits had become strong? I'd like to think so. Who knows what is possible with a healthy spirit?

The kids called their dad, who said he would come to be with them. They really seemed quite composed when he arrived. They had done so much on their own and had done it so well that I wasn't surprised to see them so courageous.

I had long before told Mary that one of us from hospice would come to the house when she died. She asked me that if her ex-husband decided to come to the house at the time of her death, would we please see to it that she looked presentable. Well, I fixed Mary's pretty hair, gave her a bath, and dressed her in her beautiful pink nightgown. I had to use bleach to clean her dentures, which had turned blue from the liquid morphine she had been taking for her pain. She was ready when her ex arrived.

As he stood with Scott and Jo-ann and looked at her, I thought, *Mary, rest in peace. Your physical and emotional pain are over.* But best of all, her spirit had survived and had become even stronger throughout her dying ordeal. Scott and Jo-ann's spirits had also survived and strengthened during this time. Watching her children become stronger and knowing that they would be okay had relieved much of Mary's anxiety. It was a gift that allowed her to die in peace.

I attended Mary's funeral. Sometimes I have a need to do that. She was such a special lady and had shared so much with me while she was dying. Both Scott and Jo-ann seemed happy to see me there. Jo-ann's boyfriend was at her side, along with Scott. Both of Mary's children gave me a big hug. They said they were so happy that their mother could stay at home with them. They were glad they could do that for her. Again, I told them how proud their mother was of them and how grateful she was for the care they had lovingly given to her. They had both matured from the experience.

To this day I am thankful that I followed my heart and went to Mary's home that final day. I haven't talked to Scott or Jo-ann in years, but when I'm driving anywhere near that street, I think of them and feel at peace. Indeed, spirits do matter!

LESSON 3

False Hope Does More Harm than Good

> Acceptance is not something an individual can choose at will. It is not like some light switch that can at will be flicked on or off. Deep emotional acceptance is like the settling of a cloud of silt in a troubled pool. With time the silt rests on the bottom and the water is clear.
>
> Michael Kerney, MD

There are spirit takers and spirit givers. The people in our present medical system are too often guilty of being spirit takers. They do this by giving false hope through futile treatments that chip away at the person who is in the body they are trying to save. Most of the time, they have no comprehension of the devastation wrought by their well-meant but misguided actions. They give you six months to live and then take it back a piece at a time by insisting on "just one more" treatment that might somehow cure the disease but succeeds only in keeping you too sick to think about anything but dying. Instead of offering false hope, appropriate end-of-life care helps us to accept what is true and gives the spirit a chance to live while there is still time. That is real hope!

What do we really need at the end of life? What kind of care should we expect? The dying deserve to be cared for in ways that celebrate and even honor their lives. It is important that this is done before they are so debilitated they have no energy to undergo this experience. To move them to this possibility, they need the loving truth from others. This is the only means they have to begin the journey that takes them beyond the suffering of their spirits. They need the help of those who are trained in this type of care.

Just as we would not have surgery without some anesthesia, I have seen that end-of-life care without hospice can be dreadful. The comfort care of the spirit afforded by hospice can add life to our days and even days to our lives. At this point, improving quality of life is far more important than delaying death. When we find out what is most important to the dying person, we also find out what will bring them hope. Just asking a person, "What do you want or need?" can be an important part of giving hope and keeping the spirit alive while that person is dying.

The false hope given by the medical profession that one more round of chemotherapy or a new experimental drug might affect a cure often robs patients of their hope for some quality of life in the short time they have left. The bad choices that are often made "in our best interests" are soon buried and forgotten, and the medical community is not held accountable for the misery it has caused in its unrelenting quest to defeat death. Physicians must have the courage to say to their patients, "There is nothing more I can do medically to cure your disease, but there is much more that can be done to help you." They must learn that there is a difference between letting go and giving up.

Margaret

When I first visited Margaret, I found a very sick woman who had been in bed for two weeks. She and her husband lived on a street of small, modest houses that all looked alike. It was one of those older, comfortable neighborhoods with well-manicured lawns and one-car garages in the back. Like Margaret, the neighborhood was past its prime. Once, I imagined, the houses were filled with children, and neighbors probably knew each other and visited frequently. But there were no children playing outside on this warm summer day. The street was very quiet.

As I parked in the driveway and was getting out of my car, Margaret's husband opened the front door. Climbing the three steps into their home, I could see the harassed look on his face. He greeted me with a smile, however, and welcomed me warmly with a handshake. He immediately took me to see his wife in their bedroom. My heart fell. She was in excruciating pain. She was weak; she had eaten very little due to the nausea and vomiting caused by the chemotherapy she was receiving. I was here because she was simply too miserable to deal with another crisis and had refused her physician's direction to take an ambulance to the hospital. Even though she was still receiving treatment for her disease, her exasperated physician, not knowing what else to do, had ordered a hospice assessment.

Margaret, or Peggy, as she preferred to be called, was sixty-seven years old. She had that twinkle in her eye that one often sees in those I fondly call "pistachio" people. Such people are not plain vanilla; they have sparkle and flavor. I could tell that underneath her illness, Peggy was one of them. I also knew that if she could find some comfort, she would be a delightful person to know.

I looked around. The bedroom was disheveled. Clothes lay on the bed, on the floor, and on top of the dresser. The bed linens, littered with used tissues, were half on and half off the bed. The room had a stale, sickroom smell. Peggy was propped up on a number of pillows but found little comfort because the pillows appeared to have been placed under her as haphazardly as the clothes had been tossed onto the floor. Worst of all, she hadn't had a bath in a week because she was too weak to get in and out of the tub.

Dale, Peggy's sixty-eight-year-old husband, was disheveled too and was exhausted from trying to take care of her. He was sad and confused and had no idea how to care for his ailing wife. He was dressed in baggy jeans held up by wide black suspenders over a wrinkled white t-shirt. His thinning white hair wasn't combed, and he looked as if he needed a shave. For most of the two and a half hours that I was there, he walked around aimlessly, wringing his hands and saying, "I don't know what to do."

I realized that my first priority was simply to inject some order and peace into this frightened, frazzled household. As I began my work, I explained everything I was doing so Dale could watch and learn. First, I cleared some of the tissues and other things out of the way and arranged the pillows to make Peggy more comfortable. Then I assessed her pain, listened to the history of her illness, took her vital signs, and gave her a physical assessment. I thought, *How sad it is that they have reached this hopelessness, this chaotic crisis stage. It doesn't have to be this bad for them.* They had needed hospice help long before this, but no one in the medical community thought to suggest it to them. Even though the treatments continued to fail and the cancer was spreading, this was the "medical care" Peggy was receiving.

After my assessment, I phoned her physician and asked him for a hospice order. I told him that Peggy had decided to stop all aggressive treatments; she did not want to live like this. I suggested that she needed stronger pain medication and a medication for her nausea and vomiting. He was happy to order all three and faxed the prescriptions to the pharmacy. I called our hospice office, and they sent a volunteer to pick up the medications and deliver them to Peggy's home.

Before I left, I gave Peggy a bath in her bed. I gave her the new medications then helped her to get comfortable. I wrote down medication instructions for Dale and promised that I would come back the next day. I assured Dale and Peggy that hospice nurses would be available to them twenty-four hours a day, seven days a week, if they had problems or questions regarding Peggy's care or Dale's concerns.

As I drove to my next patient's home, I thought about Peggy and Dale. On our initial assessment with new hospice patients, we always ask them, "What are your goals?"

Peggy had replied, "Are you crazy? I'm dying! What goal should I have?"

I told her that perhaps a first goal could be to get rid of the pain and the nausea. After that, I would ask her about her goals again. I also added, "More than you think can be possible."

In just two weeks, Peggy improved tremendously. With the nausea gone and the pain under control, she started getting out of bed and eating again. As Peggy did better, Dale did too. He had tried so hard to take care of his wife but just didn't know how and had been given no instruction. Part of my job was to teach him, and the more he learned, the stronger he became emotionally.

Now, hospice had not changed a thing about Peggy's advanced disease. It was still life limiting and progressive in nature. But as we helped her and Dale manage it, a little sunshine came back into their lives. As we in hospice see so often, when you help people feel better, they often do better. Peggy and Dale were no exception.

Our physical therapist, Helen, came to Peggy's home twice a week and helped her to regain some movement and strength. Our nurse's aide, Jan, helped with her personal care until she became strong enough to do it herself. The entire hospice team became involved in many other aspects of care for Peggy and her family.

The more Peggy could do for herself, the happier she became. Her spirit was revived. She was like a parched flower that had blossomed with just a little watering. She became more pistachio than ever! I loved visiting with Peggy and getting to know her family. Dale was so relieved to see her smiling again and enjoying life that he began to smile too. He relaxed. Best of all, their married son and daughter began visiting again and bringing their young children. They had stayed away because Peggy and Dale had insisted that they didn't want to be a burden to the family and couldn't bear to let their adult children see what was happening in their home.

Two weeks after my first visit, I arrived at their home for my regular assessment and found Peggy sitting in the living room waiting for me, dressed in regular clothes. Her hair was combed, and she didn't look as ill as before. She looked as if she were ready to go out and do errands or go to lunch with friends. As I walked in, she beamed. "Well, what do you think?"

"You look great!" I responded enthusiastically.

"No," she said, "what do you think about a goal now?" It was then that she told me that if she could, she would like to go to Florida one more time.

I replied, "Of course you can, if you have enough money!"

"Judy," she said, "I'm not going to need this money when I die, so I might as well spend it while I'm here, doing what I love to do."

I asked her if she needed her nurse to go along. We laughed together and right then began making her plans. She booked a flight for herself, her husband, their children (and spouses), and grandchildren. I arranged for a hospice in Florida to see her if she needed help while she was there. This was not a trip they could put off—Peggy was dying. I knew that these months and weeks before her death would be very precious to all of them.

One week later, they all went to the airport. They boarded her wheelchair, medications, and the other supplies she would need. Every few days for two weeks I received a postcard from Peggy. They wheeled her through Walt Disney World, EPCOT Center, and the MGM studios. She was able to see the wonderful exhibits and pavilions at EPCOT and watch her grandchildren enjoy the rides and attractions at Disney World and MGM. In the afternoons, she would sit under a tree, soaking up the warm sunshine, watching her grandchildren, Alex, Caity, and Ayden, swim.

I was so grateful that we could give that family such a pistachio time together. They made memories those weeks they will never forget. I couldn't help thinking of how bereft and hopeless Peggy and Dale had been the first time I met them. Hospice had indeed worked its miracle. Peggy hadn't been cured, but her spirit had been given new life.

Peggy was home just a few short months before cancer took her life. Before she died, however, she said the time that she had been on hospice was some of the best time in her life. Just think of the wonderful memories the members of that family have of their grandmother, mother, and wife.

When I think of Peggy I have to smile. Dale is doing well. He often said that in Peggy's final stage of cancer, before hospice, he could barely cope with his feelings of hopelessness. After hospice taught him how to care for her, he felt so much stronger. They ended their forty-eight years together as they had begun—not in a stark hospital but in their small bungalow on a comfortable street, free of pain, enjoying their life together.

LESSON 4

Hope Is Possible; It Just Changes Direction

Hope is an orientation of the spirit, an orientation of the heart. It is not the conviction that something will turn out well, but the certainty that something makes sense, regardless of how it turns out.

Vaclav Havel

Hope has two lovely daughters: Courage, so that what should be will be, and Anger, so that what should not be will not be.

St. Augustine

Dying Time—desire to live gives way to other hopes:

a. That the treatment will not be more unbearable than the disease

b. There will be an absence of pain and other symptoms

c. That caregivers will offer support to the end

Bulkin and Lukashok

Even when cure is not possible, hope is! Hope for comfort both physically and emotionally. Hope to maintain some control in the process of living while dying.

Hope and the human spirit are inseparably intertwined. Hope is an essential ingredient for maintaining a healthy spirit. Without hope, the spirit suffers and can completely collapse, resulting in deep depression and even suicide. Many times, when the dying finally realize there is no hope for curing their disease, they give up hope altogether, and their spirits also begin to die. The tragedy of a dying spirit can be reversed or even prevented in the first place by giving the dying person a new hope to hold onto. Once that new spark of hope is accepted and takes hold, the spirit is on the road to recovery.

It is widely accepted by family members, medical professionals, and many clergy that the foremost virtue in a terminally ill patient is to keep on fighting the disease and maintain to the end the hope that a cure will be achieved. Unfortunately, this notion often leads to unnecessary suffering and loss of precious time. A terminally ill person's initial hope may be only for a miraculous cure. This hope should never be taken away from them. As the reality of the situation sets in, however, other hopes become possible. What becomes most important, then, is hope that the last months, weeks, and days will be lived in comfort in the security of a home or a homelike setting, supported and loved by friends and family, with some time to make amends and to say goodbye. Equally important is the hope that the significance of one's life will be recognized.

To move us toward genuine hope, we need honesty from others about our condition, but it must be given in a sensitive manner. Hope is not accomplished by trivializing the significance of the illness, feeling sorry for us, or pretending that all will be well. Well-intentioned fabrications of the truth will not support us in our quest for hope. They serve only to enable us to remain victims of our situation.

Fear and anxiety are a constant part of the dying experience. When we learn we are not powerless, when we have named that which we fear, those fears are not as terrifying as we thought they would be. Hope then allows us to see our lives and our deaths from a different perspective. This can bring much peace and compassion to us and to all those involved. Until then, fear can paralyze and exhaust us, robbing us of hope.

Jane

Much of my hospice experience occurred while working in a hospital-based program. During that time I wore many hats, one of which labeled me as a hospital discharge planner. That is how I met Jane.

She was waiting for me when I entered her hospital room that warm sunny day in early April. We had never met before, but she knew that I was a nurse and that it was my job, with the help of hospice, to get her out of the hospital so she could go home.

Jane was in her late sixties and had just been diagnosed with metastatic pancreatic cancer. She lived in a retirement community with her much-loved dog, Sasha. She told me that her daughter, Daryl, lived nearby with her husband and two young children. Daryl worked part time as a hairdresser, but she was still able to spend a lot of time with her mother. Jane knew her cancer was incurable and had refused all of the aggressive treatments suggested by her physician. She just wanted to go home.

I was impressed with her ability to take charge and to direct her dying as she saw fit. So often, patients will let others make decisions for them and thereby lose the ability to retain even a small degree of control over their situation. This may work out if the patient's needs and wishes are being met. Far too often, however, this is not the case, and the patient is left feeling like a victim in a system that doesn't always know when to stop aggressive treatments that are ultimately futile.

Jane remained hopeful even though she knew her disease was fatal. Hope, for her, was that she would be in control and that she would be pain free in the process. She didn't even look ill that afternoon, but she knew that she was making the right decision to refuse treatments. I noticed her kind face as she greeted me pleasantly. I saw joy in her demeanor as we gently shook hands and smiled at each other. She wasn't sad, and she wasn't looking for pity. Pity was not part of the process that day or any other while she was in our care.

"Judy, I just want to go home as soon as I can," she said as I sat on her bed. "I am very involved with my group of friends in the community. I want to live my life to the very end as well as I can. I want to do my activities with my friends and family as long as I can." In fact, she was fully dressed and ready for discharge. With her long-sleeved yellow shirt and black pants, she looked as if she were on her way to do some shopping. Her bag was packed, and her gray hair was combed to perfection. She even had her makeup carefully applied.

With a big smile on her face, she said, "The sooner you get me out of here, the quicker I can resume my life. I want you to know that I am not afraid of dying. We all die." Her eyes twinkled, but then they filled with tears. "The only thing that I am afraid of is dying in pain. I know that this type of cancer can be very painful."

She wasn't looking for pity, but she was afraid. Pity so often is likened to fear. Neither pity nor fear is very helpful in keeping one's spirit alive and well. I knew that compassion, understanding, and love—without fear and pity—were all she wanted and needed from us.

I took her hand in mine and looked her in the eye. I said, "Jane, it will be the job of hospice to make sure that doesn't happen. The nurses have had advanced courses and much experience in pain management. We know what works and what doesn't work. It will be hospice's responsibility to see to it that your physician honors your wishes to be free from pain and as active as possible for as long as possible."

To cope with fear, it must be identified. It must be seen for what it really is. After all, at this stage it was only in Jane's imagination. Once we addressed her fear and dealt with it, she could let it go. She seemed to relax, and I continued. "If the nurses can't accomplish this, we will have our medical director, who is also a physician, help your physician keep you free from pain. You have my word on it."

Jane looked at me and smiled. She said, "I trust that you will do what you say. I feel much better about it now." I knew I would not be the nurse who would be visiting her regularly in her home, so I gave her my business card and told her to call me if her pain wasn't controlled.

It was critical for her to know she had an advocate, someone in her corner, so that she could go on living her life while she was dying. Fear can be a more terrible enemy than pain. If we are not afraid of dying, life can become sweeter and more satisfying. Like so many other patients with a terminal illness, she just needed someone to alleviate her fear so she could let it go. It was all Jane needed to remain hopeful.

While she was dying, Jane exemplified just how sweet life can be. For several months she lived alone with the help of hospice, her daughter, and her friends. As she had done before she became ill, she played bridge, went out to lunch, sat on her porch visiting with her neighbors, and played with Sasha. She enjoyed those months "like no other," she told the hospice team as they visited with her in her home. Her physical condition slowly deteriorated during those months, but her spirit remained alive and well.

As part of Jane's plan for living while she was dying, when she began to eat less and became weaker, she agreed to move Sasha and herself in with her daughter. This decision was her choice. As it usually happens with most of our patients who come into hospice early enough, she had accepted the gradual loss of independence that is part of the dying process. This was so important because it allowed her to maintain some control of the decisions affecting her life. As her condition changed, the hospice nurses explained what those changes meant and what she might expect to happen next. Jane and Daryl understood and appreciated this information because it gave them the luxury of planning the best use of the time remaining. With her friends often visiting her in her daughter's home, Jane was able to undertake this journey of dying with a wonderful support system and lots of love.

Hospice was there for Jane and her family every step of the way. Hospice taught Daryl how to care for her mother and how to get the support that she herself needed during the process. Our art therapist came often to work with Daryl's children. With their artwork, they were able to work through their feelings about Grandma's illness.

Jane died in her daughter's home six and a half months after I first met her. Her daughter was at her side, and her dog was on the bed next to her. Her biggest fear had been pain, but she was comfortable right up to the end. She told her hospice nurse two weeks before she died that she was more grateful for that than for anything else. She was also grateful for the love and attention her beloved dog had received from her daughter's family. She knew that Sasha had found a new and loving home.

Daryl told the hospice nurse who attended Jane's wake, "My family and I are so grateful for the love and support you all gave to Mother and us. We couldn't have done it without you."

I love telling Jane's story because it proves how peaceful and manageable the last few months of life can be. Jane personifies a good death experience. She accepted death as part of life and resolved to make the end of her life as pleasant as possible. She had refused the aggressive and in all probability, useless, treatments that had been offered. She took charge of the process and did it her way. It also eased her daughter's heart-ache to know that her mother had died exactly the way she wanted—pain free, in familiar surroundings, encircled by those who loved her, and not hooked up to machinery or medicated beyond reason.

Good end-of-life care allows us to enjoy each moment, which is really all we have left. To someone at the end of his or her life, those moments become very precious. This should be the American way. Sadly, too often it isn't.

Bette and Sam

Bette and Sam were quite the couple. They had been married for fifty-five years, had no children, and lived in a small, well-worn white bungalow in the suburbs of a large Midwestern city.

On the first day that I went to their home, as I got out of my car, I stepped into snow up to my knees. Sam was no longer able to clear the driveway, and Bette just didn't do driveways. For the rest of the winter, I kept a small shovel in my car for such emergencies.

Sam had liver cancer. The first day I met them, I knew Sam was the boss and Bette was worried about what was going to happen to her after he was gone. He was a man who was always in complete control of any situation. The only control he was losing was his battle with cancer.

Bette was a frightened little lady. Sam bossed her around, and she ran for whatever he ordered. Sam informed me that they had called hospice for her, not for him. Bette cried for most of that visit and on many of our subsequent visits. She wanted Sam to be well. She had insisted that all aggressive treatments continue, even though they both knew Sam was not getting better. At this point, the treatments had become worse than the cancer. She was so afraid that when he died she wouldn't know how to manage her life. She had never worked outside of the home and feared the time when Sam, completely in charge of it all, would leave her alone and responsible for everything, and she was terrified at the thought of it.

As their hospice nurse, I got to know both of them quite well during those months that I visited them. Bette kept herself and their home immaculate. She always had her makeup on just so. Her hair was beauty-shop fresh, and her nails were freshly manicured. She was a friendly lady with the ardor of a new friend. We had a warm feeling about each other right from the beginning.

The house, however, had not been updated in years and was in need of repair and maintenance. The decorative cornices were chipped in places. The peeling paint was evident in most of the rooms. Bette made numerous comments about this as if to apologize to me for the condition of their home.

Sam was right. Bette needed us more than he did. Her anticipatory grief was like a monster in her life. As I worked to keep Sam comfortable and as active as possible, I still spent most of my visits listening to Bette's fears and affirming the care that she was giving to Sam. She came a long way during those months that hospice cared for them. Our social worker was instrumental in encouraging Sam to teach Bette how to manage the financial aspects of living without him—she had never written a check before his illness began. As her husband became bed bound, we taught her how to care for him. We made sure she knew she could call us any time for help.

Every time I visited them, I affirmed Bette's increasing strength and positive outlook. As her fears began to subside, she began to have hope. She became stronger and more empowered. Sam was surprised at this, but as his condition worsened, he became more dependent on her. They actually became a more loving and caring couple. It wasn't so one-sided anymore. Sam was proud of his wife. It was a joy to see this wonderful woman blossom in the face of her fear of losing her husband. I watched as he became weaker and she became stronger. I saw hope, for both of them, becoming stronger.

Their journey and newfound hope were not without their setbacks, however. One that I remember quite well occurred a few days before Sam died. Bette wasn't herself when I made my visit that day. She seemed depressed and sadder than she had been on my last few visits.

I asked her if anything had happened, and she replied, "Judy, I don't know why Sam is acting this way. We've been married all these years, and in all that time he never ignored me like he has in the past two days. I've taken care of him throughout this illness, and now, half of the time, he acts as if I'm not even here. Is he angry with me? Have I done something wrong?"

"Oh, Bette," I exclaimed. "This is all part of what Sam needs to do before he dies. It's not really about you; it's about him. Let's have a cup of tea, and I'll try to explain what this is all about." So together we went to the kitchen, made our tea, and sat down.

"Sam is going through a very normal part of dying called detachment," I told her. "It isn't written up anywhere that I know of, but this is how it was explained to me when I first started in hospice. I call it the 'here and away' process.

"You see," I continued, "in order to finish his dying, Sam needs to let go of his life. When he seems to ignore you or you can't readily get his attention, his spirit is withdrawing into itself, going away to someplace to prepare for the time when his body can no longer support it. No one knows exactly what this 'away' place is, but it isn't the same as what we call a near-death experience, where people report being sent back to life after dying. Not everyone goes through this, but it happens with about half of the hospice patients I have seen. In the beginning, Sam will spend some of his time 'away' and some of it 'here,' where he will be the same Sam as always. As time goes on, he may spend more time away. This is about you only insofar as he is not yet ready to leave you, and so he keeps coming back. When he feels comfortable with being away or maybe when his body just can't bring him back anymore, he will let go of his life and die. This is the work that he will do to prepare himself for his death."

From what I have seen, detachment appears to be a peaceful process for the dying but can be quite distressing to the caregiver, who feels suddenly shut out and tends to take it personally. It was important for Bette to understand this. She was so relieved to know that Sam wasn't angry with her or disappointed in her. Knowing this restored her confidence. Once again she knew that everything would be all right.

One month after Sam died, I received a note at the office from Bette. She wanted me to know that Sam had left her a lot of money. I knew from previous conversations that he wouldn't let her spend much money while they were married. She told me she was renovating her house and that when it was done she wanted me to come and see it. She also said that the bereavement volunteer from hospice had been to see her and had called several times and that this had helped her a lot.

Five weeks later, Bette called to invite me to her home for coffee. When I arrived, I couldn't believe Bette or her house. She was joyful and so glad to see me. She had "spent a fortune," as she put it, on her home and took me on a tour to show me everything. As we sat in the kitchen having coffee together, she told me how proud she was of herself and what she had accomplished. She said Lucille (the hospice volunteer) and she had become friends. They had joined a group of widow ladies who had dinner together once a month and were planning a senior ladies' trip together out of state. They had even gone to a spa. What a difference hospice had made!

A year after Sam's death, Bette became a hospice bereavement volunteer like her friend Lucille. She continues to this day in her eighties, supporting other widows and widowers and loving the work she is doing with hospice.

Mr. Robinson

Mr. Robinson, a man in his early seventies, was dying of cancer. He knew his diagnosis and the prognosis, but "I'm not going to let it lick me" was his motto. He was a tall man of few words and spent much of his time out back in the detached garage he had converted into a workshop. His wife, on the other hand, was most often found in the house, working on her crafts. They lived in an older neighborhood where the houses lining the street all looked about the same—small, two stories, porch in front, with the driveway leading along the side of the house to the garage in the back. I always parked beside the house and entered through the side door, which went directly into the kitchen.

I visited Mr. Robinson regularly and became close to him and his wife. He wasn't big on touching and *never* hugged. One day as I was leaving, Mrs. Robinson and I were giving each other our normal good-bye hug. I reached out for Mr. Robinson and gave him what I told him was a "half a hug." He laughed and reminded me that he wasn't a hugger. I laughed back and commented that maybe he was teachable. This became the joke between the two of us. He turned out to be wonderful student of hugs. Before long he was reaching out for me as I finished my visits and giving me a hug.

The Robinsons had two adult children. Their daughter, Ilene, lived in Washington DC. She did government work, and they were very proud of her. Many times while I was there, they told me stories of their wonderful daughter. Her picture was framed and on display in several rooms in their home. I never got to meet her, and to my knowledge, she never visited them during the time that her father was on hospice.

They also had a son, Larry, who was married and lived in the area. Mr. Robinson rarely talked about his son. I often wondered about their relationship, but Mr. Robinson never brought it up. Larry visited his mother and dad in the evenings after work, so I never had a chance to meet him.

The day that Mr. Robinson died, his wife had me paged and I went to their home. When I got there, I prepared his body, called the funeral home, and went to stay with Mrs. Robinson in the kitchen. She informed me that Larry had a business trip planned and had already gone to the airport. Fortunately, we were able to contact him before he boarded the plane. I called the funeral home and asked them to wait to pick up Mr. Robinson's body until after his son could get to the home.

Mrs. Robinson and I were sitting in her kitchen when I heard a cry come through the front door. As we hurried to the living room door, I saw a large man in a shapeless brown suit.

He trembled as he sobbed. "I should have known; I should have known."

His mother took him in her arms and asked, "What should you have known?"

As she introduced us, he said, "I should have known that my dad would die today, and I should have canceled my trip."

I told him I was very surprised that his dad had died so suddenly. I had sat with him at the kitchen table just yesterday. He had been fully clothed, eating a fish sandwich, and surely didn't look or act like a man who was so close to dying.

Larry replied that he should have known because, "My dad hugged me before I left for my trip today. I can never remember a time when my dad hugged me."

About a week later, Mrs. Robinson, who had been into craft making before her husband became so ill, brought to our hospice office a glass sun reflector that she had made for us. It read *Blessed Are They Who Give Hugs.*

This is the letter I received from Larry just two weeks after his dad died.

Dear Judy,

I just wanted to thank you for the kindness and genuine caring that you gave during my dad's illness. You were such a great help to Mom many afternoons and for that we cannot express our gratitude enough. Your "hugs and praise" meant a lot to Mom and Dad. Mom was so grateful to be able to talk to you any time. You gave us encouragement and hope when we needed it most. Thanks for teaching my dad how to hug. My only regret is that I only got one, but it was enough to give me hope that our relationship would be much better in the time we had left.

God bless you and the wonderful work that you do,

Larry

LESSON 5

Silence Is Part of the Problem

A dead leaf, yellow and bright red, a leaf from the autumn. How beautiful that leaf was, so simple in its death, so lively, full of the beauty and vitality of the whole tree and summer. Strange that it has not withered ... Why do human beings die so miserably? ... Why can't they die naturally and as beautifully as this leaf?

J. Krishnamurti
Last Journal, 1987

Dying without ever addressing the issue of dying adds to the grief that dying persons and their loved ones are experiencing.

Few in our nation want to talk about death and dying, whether it is an immediate issue staring them right in the face or is off in some distant, unknowable future. The importance of talking about this matter with your family and loved ones ahead of time cannot be overstated. As you will see, never before has preemptive conversation about this crucial issue been more important. Waiting until you or a loved one is critically ill is often too late. You and I both know that life is terminal, yet you won't hear this from the mainline medical community. You won't hear this from most physicians, most hospitals or nursing homes, and most nurses. Even some clergy won't talk about "it." I hid from the ultimate truth too, until I became a hospice nurse.

The importance of good care at the end of life cannot be overstated. Most of us depend on our physicians to advise us in this situation. Yet most physicians are given little training in end-of-life care. Nor are they trained to have conversations with their patients about dying. They tend to be uncomfortable with dying and as a consequence, often avoid the subject. Modern medicine considers death as a personal defeat and will do almost anything to keep a body "alive." Physicians often have a difficult time saying, "There is nothing more that I can do to make you well." They are the experts in curing disease but far too often do us no good by prolonging our lives. Patients and families who may want to say, "Enough" are often intimidated and remain silent when pressed to go along with that one last procedure that might be the cure.

We must learn that we are not obligated to use every possible procedure or treatment that might be available. Being kept alive in the unrealistic hope that one more medication or treatment might affect a cure more often than not becomes a torture that is relieved only when death inevitably and compassionately ends the suffering. The problem is that futile, disabling treatments, when carried right up until the end, rob the dying person of any chance to regain even a semblance of spirit and dignity.

If we started talking about death and dying, we would be able to expose the amount of suffering the dying often experience. Dying is often very hard, but it should not be gruesome. If we use all of our energy, resources, and time fighting the battle—while besieged with poor symptom control, emotional denial, and aggressive futile treatments—we will not have the time or the energy to attain peace, personal growth, and closure before death occurs. Keeping silent will not protect us. So often hospice workers hear, "Why didn't anyone tell me about this wonderful program before now? I have needed this help for so long but didn't even know that I could get it."

Far too few people are offered hospice care, and for many of those, not until a crisis occurs just days or hours before death. It is usually offered in a negative statement. The message then becomes, "You are dying, and there is nothing else we can do for you."

Hospice should never mean that you are dying soon. It should mean that even though there is no cure for your terminal disease, hospice will help you live and enjoy whatever time you have left.

When cure is not possible, we need to do very little in the way of treatment for the disease. By doing very little we are actually doing a lot. It is so important to provide care for dying patients in ways that honor, support, and even celebrate their lives. We cannot do this if we are focused on the disease rather than on the person who has the disease. Patient care aside, the amount of money that would be saved by utilizing hospice instead of forcing futile care could go a long way in correcting and even saving our current health care system.

Yes, we are living longer but not necessarily better. Our senior citizens are seeing this in their own families and friends, and they are frightened that it will happen to them. As a result, they have traded their youthful fear of not living long enough to a fear of living too long, and rightly so. As if that wasn't bad enough, inappropriate end-of-life care often impoverishes the patients and their loved ones. In our nation, too many of us are financially ruined when death finally takes us. The thought of this can be devastating to the one who is ill and adds to the pain of the spouse who is left behind. The enemy, then, is not death but ignorance, fear, and denial. From what I have seen, being under-informed and undereducated are the worst things that can happen to us when we become terminally ill. If we are to have some control of our deaths, we need to break down the wall of silence and talk about dying before the fact.

David

I first met David early on a Saturday morning when I was on call for our hospice program. He was an eighty-one-year-old gentleman with terminal cancer. His wife, Eleanor, an elderly, frail woman, was trying her best to take care of David at home. I remember how tired she looked that day.

Her short gray hair was swept off of her face with an old-fashioned hairnet. The sparkle, if there ever was one, was gone from her eyes. Her body was bent over, but she was doing her best to help her husband. She told me that David had been in and out of the hospital many times during the past two years trying to fight this "terrible cancer." Their funds were diminishing, and both of them were exhausted from worry and frustration. His cancer and the treatments he was receiving had taken their toll on both of them. She said that she had seen an article about hospice in the newspaper and wondered if we could help them. They had had a very difficult night and requested that I come to their home as soon as possible. I was there in less than an hour.

I found David sitting in his chair, crying in pain. He was thin and sallow. I sat on an easy chair across from him, wondering how could he have gotten to this stage without somebody (like his physician) doing something. His voice cracked as he told me that he had been in pain all night but didn't want to go to the hospital "ever again." He begged me to help him. I quickly assessed the situation and telephoned his physician, who, fortunately, gave me an order for hospice care. He asked that I call him back as soon as I had done a complete evaluation.

As so often happens, this became crisis management instead of hospice care. I spent three hours at David's home getting the necessary equipment brought in and getting pain medication ordered, delivered, and given to David.

I learned a lot about David and Eleanor that day. They had been married fifty-six years and had lived in the same tiny old home all of that time. They had no children or family in the area, but they did have a wonderful old dog that was David's best friend. They had never talked with each other about David's worsening condition, nor had their physician discussed this with them. They felt that they were stuck in this situation with little choice in the matter.

I looked at this tiny little lady and remembered two families I had worked with during that past year. The elderly spouses were so depleted by the time hospice was called that they, the caregivers, died before the hospice patients did. None of these families had made any plans for the eventual last stage of the patient's disease. As it happened with David, they hadn't talked about it with their physician or with anyone else, it seemed. After I explained hospice to both of them, Eleanor asked in both frustration and amazement, "Why didn't anyone tell us about hospice? This is just the help that we've been looking for."

Toward the end of our visit, David said to me, "Judy, would you like to meet the most wonderful dog in the whole world?" Of course, I said I would love to.

Eleanor took me to the kitchen and down three steps to the door leading to the backyard. In a yard overgrown with weeds, we found Ben, an aging collie, tied to a dog run. His face was gray with age, and his eyes were clouded with cataracts, but his spirit was alive and well. With a wagging tail he came to us. Eleanor let him into the house, and he tried to go up those three steps but just couldn't make it. She lifted Ben's arthritic back legs up the stairs, and off he went to find his best friend. David smiled from ear to ear as Ben took his place beside his master.

For the rest of my visit, David kept his hand on Ben's head or patted his back. The love between the two of them was obviously deep and had a long history. By the time I left that day, I knew that David was comfortable and that Eleanor was not only given instruction on how to take care of her husband but that she felt supported in his care. She knew that I or another nurse from hospice was but a telephone call away.

David was on our program for the next three weeks. For the first week he was still able to get out of bed and walk to the living room. As he became unsteady on his feet, we ordered a walker for his safety and to make it easier for Eleanor to help him. Our physical therapist came several times to show them how to use the walker. As David became weaker, the therapist taught Eleanor how to get him in and out of bed and into a chair.

Once hospice was involved, David spent his final time in complete comfort in his home with his loving wife and his best friend, Ben, at his side. Both Eleanor and David understood that it was time to treat David, not the disease that he had, which was by then untreatable. The more they learned and understood, the less frightening it became for them.

I made numerous visits to their home during the next three weeks. Eleanor and David appeared to enjoy the time they spent together. Eleanor looked rested and much less stressed even though David's condition was worsening. This was typical with our hospice families. As patients become more terminal, more often than not their care becomes easier. The patient sleeps more, eats less (if at all), and does not require as much hands-on care.

To help Eleanor, a hospice volunteer would take her shopping and to get her hair done while another volunteer stayed with David so she would not worry about being gone. This was important "medicine" for Eleanor's spirit. All the effort she had given to David's care had drained her, so we did all that we could to help fill her up and renew her spirit.

Caregivers need this replenishment to do their best care giving. You can't give away what you don't have to give.

The financial burden of David's illness had been almost too much for them. Now the medications that had used up so much of their social security were paid for by hospice. Our social worker, Kathy, helped to sort out the bills that had been collecting over the time David had been ill. Eleanor had been overwhelmed by all of this and just didn't know where to begin to face this mountain of paperwork. David had been worried that Eleanor would lose their home due to so many unpaid bills. Kathy helped them find the agencies that would provide the assistance they needed to keep this from happening. Yes, much of their savings and other resources had been used up, but now they both were confident that Eleanor would continue to have a place to live and enough money to live on.

As she had been instructed, Eleanor called early one morning to tell me that David had died. I told her I would be there as soon as I could get dressed and drive to her home. She assured me that she would be fine until I got there. She said that when she woke up that morning she had found Ben sitting beside David's bed with David's hand resting on Ben's head. Eleanor wasn't sure when David had died, but Ben had stayed beside him until Eleanor woke up.

When I arrived at their home forty-five minutes later, I found Ben lying on the floor beside David. As I prepared David's body for the funeral home to pick up, Ben stayed in the room with me. I have often been impressed with the love from the animals when I go to the home when someone has died. Ben was no exception.

When David's body was ready for the funeral director, Ben and I went to comfort Eleanor. She told me she was so grateful that her family (the three of them) had the opportunity to remain at home together the last three weeks of David's life. She said David told her that knowing she wouldn't lose their home was most comforting for him. Most important for her was that David had died in complete comfort with his best friend at his bedside.

Lynda

Lynda lived in a small three-bedroom home with Robert, her husband of thirty-five years. Their home was a one-story redbrick dwelling on a busy street of other homes just like theirs. A creek ran through the development, adding appeal to the area. They were both only in their fifties.

Robert, a balding, slender, medium-height businessman, met me at the door and led me into a small, neat living room, where I met his family. I found two neatly dressed young women seated on the edge of a couch. He introduced them as his daughters, who were both nurses at the hospital where Lynda was first diagnosed with cancer. Liz and Sandie knew how ill their mother was but dealt with it by not acknowledging it. Neither had much experience with death or dying in the orthopedic units where they worked.

They all impressed me as warm, caring, and down-to-earth people. After we talked for a while, the three of them took me in to meet Lynda. She was curled up in a twin-sized bed. She was a tiny woman who greeted me with a weak smile. She managed an occasional nod as I explained hospice to the four of them.

When I visited the home, I usually found Robert in the kitchen with his daughters; most of the time all three had been crying. I talked with them to find out how they were coping with Lynda's illness and her care. Both girls knew how to give their mother her nursing care—this was not a concern. However, they said they were having such a hard time keeping Lynda from knowing how sick she was. They couldn't cry in front of her, or "she would know."

Then I would go to the back bedroom where Lynda was confined in bed, and she would tell me that she knew she was very ill, but her husband and daughters didn't know how sick she was. She didn't want them to know. What a heartbreaking situation; Lynda was dying alone while her family stayed in the kitchen. I tried to help them understand that she needed them, but they were too frightened to face what was happening. The entire family knew that I was from hospice but didn't want to admit to themselves what that meant.

Lynda's physician had never told her that she was dying. He just sent hospice out there without an explanation, expecting us to tell her. This information was not a surprise to me. Often, physicians won't tell their patients the truth about a terminal illness. They say they don't want them to give up hope. I have strongly disagreed with this. Just because the intention is good, it doesn't justify the action. To send a nurse from hospice out to a home without being truthful with the patient and loved ones is, in my estimation, an injustice. I have had families say to me that they looked up the word *hospice* in the dictionary just to make sure they understood why I was coming to their home. A physician's reluctance in being truthful often causes more harm than good. It certainly did in this home.

With each visit, I found a growing sadness in Lynda. One day she seemed especially depressed. Taking a moment to collect myself, I said to her, "Lynda, what do you think is happening to you?"

She answered, "I think that I'm dying. What do you think?"

I said, "I think you are right. Wouldn't you rather do this with the love and support of your family than to be so all alone back here in your bedroom?"

She replied, "Yes, it's very lonely, and I get scared when I think about it."

I told her that her family felt the same way. I asked her if she would mind if I told them how she felt, and she said, "Oh, Judy, if you would, I would be so grateful." Then she asked me why her physician hadn't told her that she was dying.

I asked her if she had any idea why, and she ventured a guess. "I don't know for sure, but I think that he is probably more afraid of death than I am." I laughed and said that there was more truth to that than even she and I could believe.

I went out to the kitchen and told Robert that Lynda needed him and the girls as much as, if not more than, she ever did. I repeated the words that Lynda had said to me; then I asked all of them to be truthful with themselves and with Lynda. I told Robert that what I would want if I were dying would be for my husband to hold me and comfort all of us. "It's not good to be isolated from each other. Being separated at this difficult time is very lonely and adds to everyone's distress."

He said, "Do you mean that I can get into bed and hold my wife?" That was exactly what I meant.

I explained that there was necessary suffering and unnecessary suffering. They all will share the necessary—grief, fear, letting go. But the unnecessary—lack of connection to each other, denial of what was happening, unmanaged pain, and other symptoms—could be alleviated by them coming together with the help of hospice. I also explained the importance of completing the message of love before it is too late.

With that, I wrote down, as I did with so many loving families, the five things that must be said to complete a relationship before death. Those five things are:

1. I forgive you
2. Forgive me
3. Thank you
4. I love you
5. Goodbye

The three of them headed back to the bedroom. Many tears were shed, but there were also laughter and sighs of relief. None of them could believe that the short time they had left could be so precious.

Lynda's condition actually improved over the next few weeks. It was a surprise to all of them. I explained that when your spirit is being nurtured, your body knows it. Lynda's certainly did! Liz and Sandie told me that they were so impressed with their mother at this time in her life. They said they always knew they had a wonderful mother but that somehow, now she was more loving and accepting. She had become more of who she really was. In the words of Fred Rogers, the late children's television personality, "Anything that can be mentioned can be managed."

Most people need their loved ones with them as they are dying. This affords the opportunity to create moments of profound meaning in the lives of all involved. When we ignore reality or pretend that nothing is happening, we also lose the opportunity to give the gift of significance to the occasion. When we can acknowledge that what is happening is awful, sad, and frightening, it becomes more real and allows us to live through it and come out better for having done so. Often, this anticipatory grieving enables us to better handle the death of our loved one when that death finally happens.

Dying can be a precious time of growth for both the patient and the family. The patient is supported and not denied what he or she knows to be true, and the family gets a head start on dealing with the inevitable sorrow that comes with losing a loved one. When death does occur, much grief has already been processed, and the immediate impact is often lessened for everyone concerned.

That is exactly what happened in that loving home. As they prepared for Lynda's death, they all began to live more fully. Lynda shared her womanly wisdom with her daughters. They shared family stories and also individual stories that reflected only their own personal experiences as wife, husband, and daughters. Lynda and her family learned not to be afraid of tears—hers or theirs.

There were no regrets after Lynda died. The family had come together and helped each other through this difficult time. They were prepared and ready for death to come. With love and care, together they accomplished what none of them could have done alone. Breaking the silence had given them the time and the energy to prepare for Lynda's death. Together they had planned her funeral, wherein Lynda selected her clothes, her casket, and the songs she wanted sung. It was a healing experience for all of them.

Lynda died two months later with her daughters and her husband at her side. I later received this note from Robert.

Dear Judy,

Thank you very much for all the help and support you gave to my family and me. Most of all, that you genuinely cared. These past months were the darkest days of my life, but I have peace in my heart and mind that I did everything that I could do for my wife.

I shared her life and I was privileged to share even her death. Because of people like you, the ordeal was more bearable and your guidance and care was very much appreciated.

I can never thank you enough. You really made the difference and opened my eyes to things that the doctors never explained. Thank you so very much.

With much gratitude and affection from the girls and me,

Robert

LESSON 6

The Truth Will Set You Free

Viewing life from the prospective of death, we are made freer. Seeing something for the last time is nearly as good as seeing it for the first time.

Peter Noll
In the Face of Death, 1987

Once we face the fact that there is no cure for our disease, we can move on to completing our lives. Good medical practitioners then change their treatment focus from the disease to the person who has the disease. This places value on who we are as persons, not just as bodies that need medical attention. We can have physical comfort, set some goals that are important to us, and work toward emotional and spiritual peace.

Death is a mystery, but dying should not be. What are we hiding from? There is no power in being a victim. We should be able to come to the end of life knowing that we are valuable human beings, that our lives had meaning, and that our loved ones have also been supported in their time of need.

With the advances in medical technology, it is now possible in many cases to delay death for weeks, months, or even, in some cases, years. In our increasingly technical and secular society, this obsession with delaying death can become more important than the quality of the life that is being prolonged. When faced with the reality of a terminal illness, we often try to make believe it is not happening by distracting ourselves with the innumerable tests and treatments now available through modern medicine. We remain in denial even though, in our heart of hearts, we know the truth.

If we are to deal with the truth, however, we must first stop trying to deny it. Otherwise, we remain confused victims in a society that fears death and pressures us to extend the time of life regardless of the quality of that life. Even so, some may still choose to protect their spirits through denial, and if that is their choice, it should be accepted. However, when life is extended for no other reason than to delay death, the spirit often begins to die long before the body does. And if the spirit is dying, the person is dying—not physically, but inside.

If dying is not something to be feared, then life can become sweeter and more satisfying. This realization can bring peace and compassion to all those involved. Unfortunately, we often disregard the emotional and physical suffering caused by futile attempts to beat death and continue to struggle in an unrealistic hope for a medical cure. What does this gain? Death will come regardless. It can come with the bitterness of defeat, or it can come with the peacefulness of acceptance.

Even though praised and admired by some, stubborn determination can be an illness in itself and can add to the pain and anxiety that are already present. The dying, and in particular those around them, must understand that letting go at the proper time is not the same as giving up. Not just the medical community but also the loved ones need to ask, "Is this aggressive treatment being done for the good of the patient, or is it being done to fulfill my own need?"

Marty

Marty was a sixty-two-year-old man who lived with his wife, Lila, and their daughter, Lisa. They were the kind of people one likes almost immediately. They welcomed me into their home on that first day even though they knew my presence meant that Marty's disease was not going to be cured. They had already accepted the truth of Marty's dying. This made my job easier in that they could now focus on making good use of Marty's remaining time. I remember thinking as I walked up their front steps, *What a nice home.* The lawn was well kept, and there were flowers blooming all around the front porch.

Lisa answered the front door with a pleasant smile on her face but apprehension in her eyes. As I smiled and introduced myself, she began to cry. Thus began our relationship. I also met Marty and Lila that first day.

Marty's cancer was in his gall bladder and had metastasized throughout his abdomen. He was tall and thin, a sickly-looking man, but with a wonderful, warm smile. Lila was an attractive middle-aged woman who graciously welcomed me into their home. She appeared to have things under control but was grateful for some extra help in caring for her husband. They had just celebrated their fortieth wedding anniversary, and Marty had to show me all of the many cards of congratulations they had received.

Lisa was about thirty-five years old; pretty, with a slim figure, dark hair, large, intelligent brown eyes, and a warm, contagious laugh. She was single and worked full time in an office. She appeared to have a close relationship with both of her parents. Marty and Lila also had a son who lived about three hundred miles from them with his wife and two young children. Ron and Fran often drove in for the weekend, especially as Marty's condition became worse. They were a loving family, but all suffered with the knowledge of Marty's limited life expectancy.

That first visit, besides the normal paperwork and assessment, I focused on controlling the frequent bouts of pain that Marty was experiencing. Once we were able to get his pain and other symptoms managed, he was able to drive again. When I called to make my appointments to see them, he and Lila would sometimes be out for a ride or at a movie. I was always happy when that happened because it meant that Marty was having a good day.

Marty and Lila were both active in their community. Church work was important to them, as were their bowling and card groups. When Marty could no longer handle the weight of his bowling ball, he went to watch and keep score for Lila and their friends. Through their activities, they were able to maintain the company and support of their friends throughout much of Marty's illness. They had accepted the inevitable and together, with the gentle support of our hospice team, were able to live their lives making every day count. They wisely used their time concentrating on living, not dying.

Marty was on our hospice program for four months. During that time he and his family often expressed how grateful they were for all the support and care that hospice was giving them. As we taught Lila how to irrigate his biliary tubes and how to change the dressings on his abdomen, she worked through her fears and became empowered with the ability to help her husband. We instructed not only Marty but also the entire family on how to manage his pain and other symptoms so that he was comfortable yet still alert enough to enjoy their time together.

Much of our hospice work with Marty and his family involved teaching and patient care, but many times our visits were spent just talking about life and death and the concerns that were most important to all of them. Marty's deepest fear, he told me, had been that he would have to go back into the hospital and that perhaps he would die there. Now he knew that with hospice help he would be able to remain at home until the end.

Marty's condition took a sharp decline about three weeks before he died. We made frequent visits to their home during that time, along with much telephone support. We answered calls in the middle of the night and did late visits when necessary. Our home health aide began making visits to help Lila with Marty's personal care. She taught Lila how to bathe and turn Marty and even how to change the bed linens while he was still in the bed. We maintained close contact with all of the family during this critical time. Ron often called me long distance at my office for updates on his father's condition and to get my gut feeling about how his mother and sister were doing.

I was on forty-eight-hour call when Lila had me paged on a Saturday morning. She told me that Marty's pain was worse and asked if I would please come to their home. When I arrived, I saw a definite change in Marty's condition from my visit just the day before. I placed a call to his physician to bring him up to date on what was happening and to ask for more pain medication. He insisted that I get an ambulance and have Marty brought to the hospital. When I told this to Lila and Marty, they both refused, saying that he wanted to stay at home and be kept comfortable. It took three more calls to Marty's physician before he agreed to adequate pain control.

I finally had to say, "Marty is dying. The only thing that he wants is to remain in his own home with his family and to be comfortable. I am on call for the next twenty-four hours, and I am not leaving here until he *is* comfortable and his family is okay. I can call you every five minutes until then, or you can agree to give the medication he needs with this call." He finally agreed then to order what Marty needed to control the pain.

At this point, Lila said she really needed to get some fresh air. Both she and Marty had been up much of the night trying to deal with the changes in his condition. Lisa was at work, so Lila asked if I would stay with her husband while she went to pick up the newly ordered medication.

Even though Marty wasn't very comfortable, he had something that he wanted and needed to do before he died. He was very weak and hardly able to speak by this time. He was, however, able to point and make his requests clear to me. This frail, dying man wanted a pen, some paper, and his reading glasses. I propped him up in bed and placed the pen in his hand, his glasses on his nose, and bent his knees to rest the paper on his legs so he could proceed to write a short "love letter" to each member of his family. The one that I remember the most was to his daughter-in-law, Fran.

> Dear Fran,
>   The Blue Nun is in the cabinet in the basement. Have one for me.
>   I love you,
>
> > > Dad

Between letters he would drift off then shake his head and have me set him up again so that he could write. One time I said to him, "Marty, are the angels coming for you each time you close your eyes?" He looked at me with a grateful smile, as though he was glad that someone understood. He nodded his head yes. I replied, "You're not ready for them yet, are you?" He shook his head no.

Just after Lila got back from the pharmacy, Ron and Fran arrived. By then Marty had finished writing the four letters that were so important to him. His pain was becoming worse, and I said to him, "Marty, your vital signs are changing. When I give you this medication, you might fall asleep and not wake up. Are you ready for that possibility?" With a slight smile on his face, he shook his head no. Then this very courageous man, still in severe pain, held out his hands.

The four of us held hands with him around his bed as he began to mouth, and together we joined him in saying the Lord's Prayer. One by one he kissed everyone goodbye. He pointed his finger at me; I kissed him on the cheek and whispered in his ear, "I'll see you in heaven." With that familiar twinkle in his eye and the sense of humor that I had come to love, he crossed his fingers and pointed to me as if to say, *I don't know if you will make it!*

I smiled and said, "Marty, are you ready for your pain medication now?" He nodded his head yes. There wasn't a dry eye in the room, including mine, but everyone understood. The next day Marty died. Lila said that he was awake off and on and very comfortable.

Marty died in his home, with his family by his side, right where he wanted to be, with the care and control that he deserved. When I went to the visitation at the funeral home, his family said that they were so grateful for the time that they were able to take care of Marty. They especially treasured their love letters.

It has been my privilege to work with many wonderful people who, after the truth is known and accepted, spend the end of their lives in ways that are meaningful and important to them. As strange as it may seem to those who haven't experienced it, the dying of a loved one can be a very sacred time in the life of a family.

LESSON 7

No One Should Have to Live Dying in Pain

We all must die. But that I can save him from days of torture, that is what I feel as my great and ever new privilege.

Albert Schweitzer

From what I have seen, nothing destroys a spirit more than poorly treated pain. Pain is a medical emergency and a frightening enemy! Physical pain in the life of a terminally ill patient exists either because physicians aren't educated in good pain management or because they just don't try. Many in the medical community already know how to manage physical pain. The solutions are readily available to remedy this human, social, and medical disgrace of dying in pain, robbed of any chance for a useful life in the time that is left.

Medications and techniques well known to the hospice community can completely control pain in all but a small fraction of patients. What prevents us from availing ourselves of these solutions? Why are so few of our people provided with good pain management when facing a life-limiting illness? In recent years the medical community has attempted to correct this, but it still remains a major problem to those who are dying. If this crime against humanity is ever going to be stopped, we can't continue to look away and pretend that it is not happening. The only answer is to acknowledge that this terrible "care" occurs, stop accepting it, and change it!

Billie

It was about eleven a.m. on a cold spring day when Esther, our hospice manager, came to my desk. Urgently, she said, "Judy, there is a family in your town that I just spoke to on the phone. They are in a crisis and need some help now!"

As I quickly put on my coat, Esther told me what Kimm, the young woman who called, had told her. Kimm's mother, Billie, (age sixty-four) had been in the hospital for the past two weeks following the surgery during which her terminal cancer was discovered. She had been sent to her daughter's home to recover from the surgery and to stay there until she died. Esther said she could hear Billie in the background crying out in pain as she talked to Kimm. In despair, Kimm cried, "My mother is in so much pain, and I don't know what to do! I called her doctor, and he told me to give her the medication he had ordered plus some Tylenol. He said to expect her to be in a lot of pain—she is, after all, dying of cancer."

Her mother refused to go back to the hospital. Kimm was scared and tired (they both had been up all night) and was crying on the phone. She had called the home care nurse who had taken care of her dad, who had died just three months before. The nurse had advised her to call hospice for help.

Even though it was rush hour, the traffic was light. As I drove the twenty miles to Kimm's home, I grew frustrated. This is the same sad and awful story that we in hospice hear so often: "If there isn't a way to cure you, then there isn't anything else we can do." Far too many physicians think this way, and their terrified patients accept it without question. They don't know that there is an alternative to the suffering they are enduring.

Kimm met me at the door; her pale blue eyes were red from crying. She was a young woman in her thirties who looked very thin in her gray cotton sweat suit. Her dark blond hair was uncombed, and she looked as if she hadn't slept in several days. Fear and anxiety were written all over her face, but at least for the moment, she seemed to have her emotions under control. She led me to the room where her mother was, but she didn't have to. All I had to do was follow the sound of Billie wailing in pain; I had heard it the moment Kimm opened the front door.

Billie sat in an overstuffed chair, bent over with pain, her ample body dressed in a rumpled blue and white cotton robe. Even through her misery, the assertiveness was apparent in the line of her jaw. As I approached her, the first thing she said to me as her voice cracked was, "I don't care if you call Dr. Kevorkian, just please *do something* about this pain. I can't live like this." Then she threw up.

As Kimm and I cleaned her up, Billie declared that she absolutely would not go back to the hospital. "They won't help me there," she cried. In silence, I agreed with her. The pain was something that she couldn't describe. It was sadistic what was happening to this woman.

I called her physician to ask for a hospice order and an order for appropriate pain medication. He said the same thing to me that he had said to Kimm: "She could expect to be in pain because she is dying of cancer." Knowing what I knew about pain management, I felt his statement was at least a breach of medical ethics if not just incredible ignorance. I could hear the anger in his voice as he responded to my request and hung up the phone on me. I called him back with the same request. This time, before he could hang up, I asked him if he would give me an order for hospice for Billie and let me work with our hospice medical director for medication orders. His reluctant agreement was all I needed! He was relieved of responsibility, and now we could do something about Billie's suffering.

I was greatly encouraged. I knew that now Billie would find some comfort. I called our medical director and explained the circumstances. I gave him all the information I had, including the physical assessment I had made. Over the phone, I reviewed Billie's medical records with him and asked for several orders—something for pain and something for nausea and vomiting. He agreed to this course of treatment and also sent a volunteer from hospice to pick up the medications so that Kimm and I could stay with Billie. He talked to Kimm and told her that he would come to her house the next day to see her mother.

I administered the medications as soon as they arrived, and within three hours Billie's pain had greatly subsided. In the meantime, I learned that Billie had not had a bowel movement in ten days! Not only did she have a body full of cancer but of stool as well. I thought, *How could she have been discharged from the hospital without even having a bowel movement following surgery? That's supposed to be standard procedure.* We spent most of the next three days dealing with this problem alone. This was just the beginning of the work that we would do to help her recover from this shocking excuse for medical care.

As I assessed the situation and comforted both Kimm and her mother, I listened to their story. I learned that three weeks prior to this, Billie had been mowing her grass when she experienced a severe pain in her side. She hadn't been feeling well during her husband's illness and eventual death and assumed that she was just worn out and grieving. The pain, however, continued and became too severe to ignore, so after finishing the lawn she phoned her physician, who told her to meet him at the emergency room. She was admitted to the hospital, where surgery revealed an inoperable pancreatic cancer that had already metastasized. After two weeks in the hospital, she had been taken to Kimm's home to die.

Kimm was the youngest of Billie's five adult children. She lived with her husband, Lynn, whom I met when he came home from work during my first visit. He looked to be in his thirties—a tall, thin man with boyish looks and an easy, laid-back manner. Lynn had lost his first wife to cancer. Kimm and Lynn had been married just a few months. They were wonderful with Billie, but they needed help. Billie's other children all lived within a thirty- to forty-five-minute drive from Kimm's home. They were close enough to be of help but not close enough to relieve Kimm of some of the day-to-day care.

My heart went out to this family. They had just buried their dad three months earlier, and now their mother was quite suddenly terminally ill. Not only was Billie very sick, but she felt guilty because Lynn and Kimm would start out their new life together taking care of her. All of Billie's children called the hospice office asking what they could do for their mom. They all made regular trips to Kimm's house to bring food and flowers and to sit on the porch and cry.

Only one of Billie's children was missing—the youngest son, Randy, who refused to come to Kimm's house. He and Kimm had not spoken in three years. The family said little about this except that Kimm and Randy had had a fight and that they were both stubborn. This added to Billie's emotional burdens.

Billie asked me to meet with all of her children to explain her illness and to see if they would work out a schedule to help Kimm and Lynn take care of her. Mothers are like that. Billie also told me about some fighting going on among all of her children, not just Kimm and Randy. She thought that most of the conflict was about her home and who was going to get what when she was gone.

We set up a meeting at Kimm and Lynn's home for eight p.m. on the Monday following the first week that Billie was with hospice. Everyone, even Randy, was there. I had called him myself and told him that his mom had especially wanted him to be there. At her request, Billie stayed in her bed in the other room while we met. The mood in the room was palpably tense as we introduced ourselves.

As we sat around Kimm and Lynn's dining room table, I was struck by the wishes of these children to help. Concern flooded their eyes. They all wanted to know, "What can I do?"

I said, "Your mom wants to stay at Kimm's house, but she would like all of you to help Kimm take care of her. Kimm will take a leave of absence from work, but she and Lynn would like to get out alone once or twice a week. Someone needs to stay with your mom so they can go out. Your mom also needs to see all of you being kind to each other."

I told them that I had adult children also and that nothing made me happier than seeing them happy and together, enjoying each other. I said, "If you want to really help your mom and show her how much you love her, let her see you loving and helping each other get through this difficult time." Kimm and Randy looked at each other—I mean really looked at each other—said nothing, and then looked back at me. I liked what I saw.

Next, we talked about the furnishings, pictures, and other "things" at Billie's home. I shared with them what Billie had told me. They agreed to let their mom decide how to divide up her possessions. I sat back and listened as they talked together and decided as a group how they would help Kimm. They cried a little, laughed a little, hugged (even me), and then went into Billie's room.

It was a long day for me, but many hospice days are like that. It was almost ten p.m. when the meeting broke up, but all of us, including Billie, knew that the bumpy path to her death had become a little smoother. A light rain was falling as I drove home. I was emotionally drained but pleased that everything had gone so well.

I met with Kimm and Lynn the next day to find out what their other needs were in order to keep Billie in their home. It was a small house, and there weren't many options. Hospice had put a hospital bed in their family room for Billie. Kimm had been sleeping on the floor beside her mom each night in case she needed something. We were able to solve this problem by putting a baby monitor in their upstairs bedroom so they could hear Billie if she needed them during the night. Now Kimm and Lynn could be together at night and not have to worry about Billie. This simple solution was of enormous help.

I am proud and happy to say that Billie lived—and I mean lived—for three solid months. Her pain was under control, her vomiting diminished, and her bowels were semi-functioning. She and Kimm and the others visited, shared stories of their lives, and wove sweet, new, wonderful memories together. Billie had lots of other company; grandchildren, neighbors, and friends came. Her mailman even drove twenty miles each way to see his friend Billie, to whom he had delivered mail for twenty-five years.

My patients often inspire me, and this family was no exception. What a wonderful woman Billie was. She often told me that these long summer days and nights were a treasure for her. She told me how one night they all sat together on the porch, eating hoagies from the deli (her favorite meal). That was when they all planned her funeral. Amid laughter and tears they called it the "last supper."

Once a week, Kimm or one of her siblings drove their mother to her home, where Billie placed a sticker bearing the name of a child or grandchild on the various pieces of furniture, appliances, dishes, and other items that she wanted to pass along. One day she called me at the office to say, "Judy, I'm so happy. I just marked the last thing—a potato peeler." We laughed, and I was so grateful that this large project was complete because Billie was getting weaker and didn't have much energy left. She told me her last job was to sell her house and see that everyone in her family got their fair share of the profits. Billie met with the realtor on Tuesday, and her home sold on Sunday. With her goals accomplished, she died the following Saturday.

I was the nurse on call the day Billie died. When I got to Kimm's home, all five of Billie's children were there. Three of them and Lynn greeted me outside as they sat on the front porch. They assured me they were all okay. I had called them from my car phone to tell them I was bogged down in traffic and reduced to inching forward in fits and starts; it had taken me over an hour to get there.

As I let myself in the front door, I saw Kimm and Randy sitting beside Billie's bed. Kimm told me that Randy had stayed up all night sitting with his mom so that Kimm could get some sleep. Not only were they talking to each other, but they were looking out for each other. What a blessing that Billie had seen their mended relationship.

Kimm got up from her chair, took my hand, and led me to her mom's bedside. She said, "Judy, look at my mom's face. She looks so peaceful, almost like she's sleeping and just having a nice dream. That's how she died. She just fell asleep and didn't wake up." Indeed, she did. What a difference from the first day I saw her.

Kimm continued, "Do you remember the first day you came here? How terrified my mom and I were? Do you remember how my mom's face looked then? And look at her now. Oh, Judy, thank you for all that you did for all of us but especially for my mom." With that, she picked up a figurine of an angel that had sat on the windowsill beside Billie's bed. Many times during our visits together, Billie would mention that she knew her angel on the windowsill was watching over her and taking care of her. With that, Kimm turned the figurine over, and on the bottom was a sticker with *Judy* written on it.

I still have that angel. It sits on my bookcase as a reminder to me of this wonderful, caring woman who touched my life. Sometimes I just look at it for inspiration. Thank you, Billie, for your gift to me.

Theirs is a wonderful hospice story but not an unusual one. Families do come together, so often as a result of hospice intervention. Pain can be managed. People can die in peace and in comfort. Spirits can remain alive and well even when the body is dying. This is the letter that Kimm wrote to me shortly after her mother died.

> *Dear Judy,*
>
> *I just wanted to thank you for the wonderful care you provided to my mother and for all of the help and support you provided to my family.*
>
> *It was the most difficult time in my life that I can remember, but you made it as easy to bear as possible. You do wonderful work. I am grateful that you are in the world to help others pass from this life into heaven with as little suffering as possible, focusing on life rather than death. You will always have a special place in my heart.*
>
> *With much gratitude and love,*
>
> *Kimm*

Simon

Simon and Sue weren't what I would call close, personal friends of my husband and me. Simon was the captain of the tennis team my husband, Roger, played on. When the team won the district tournament, most of the wives went out of town with the team to the state title event. Many of the wives were also tennis players, and we all had a wonderful time together. That's when I got to know Sue. She was a portly, pleasant lady who, even though she didn't play tennis, fit right in with the rest of us.

Simon loved his tennis. The men on the team respected him and enjoyed being around him. He was a nice guy, and we all appreciated his great sense of humor. He had played tennis for years, and along with golf and fishing, it was still a very important part of his life. He was reported to have been quite an athlete during his high school days, but at age sixty, Simon was overweight, not as quick as he used to be, but still an excellent tennis player. It was clear to those who knew him that Simon loved the game, but more importantly, he loved people.

Even though the team didn't win that event, we spent the weekend getting to know each other better and enjoying the friendships that were growing. That weekend was the beginning of my relationship with Simon and Sue as a couple.

Two years had passed when Simon announced at the regular Monday night men's tennis league that he was retiring and that he and Sue were moving to their summer hideaway. Their cottage home was in the woods near a lake about an hour and a half away from the tennis club where we all played. Simon's plan was to drive in each Monday night for the men's league. The guys were pleased that they would still see Simon once a week and not lose his companionship.

The following winter, Roger came home one Monday night after the league and said that he was concerned about Simon. His color was poor, he was losing weight, and he just didn't have the energy he normally had. The next week, Simon announced that he had colon cancer. We were all upset by this revelation, but Simon assured us that a leading physician was caring for him in one of the finest institutions in the nation.

The next two years were simply awful for Simon and Sue. In the beginning, every step forward in his treatment was met with two steps backward. From major infections to complications from every aspect of treatment, Simon had one setback after another.

The next news we received was that Sue also had been diagnosed with colon cancer. We tried as a group to support the two of them emotionally. Fortunately, Sue's treatment was successful, and she was on her feet and going again in a relatively short time.

Unfortunately, Simon continued to have one medical problem after another, but he finally began to see some improvement. The surgery to remove the tumor had apparently been successful, but additional operations were required to repair his damaged colon. That wasn't about to stop Simon. He was bound and determined to get back on the tennis court and the golf course—and he did. He wasn't quite the same Simon as before, but he was happy to be back and looked forward to regaining his old form.

For a while everything was looking better. Blood tests came back negative, and he seemed to be getting stronger, but it didn't last very long. The cancer came back, and this time it was inoperable.

The last time Roger and I visited him in the hospital, he was in a lot of pain. His voice was raspy and quiet as he said, "The doc told me this morning to get my affairs in order. I don't have much time left." Even though he was very sad, he agreed that he was tired of fighting a losing battle. He knew I was a hospice nurse and asked me if I would help Sue to understand. I told him I was willing and able to help in any way they needed. He thanked me, kissed me goodbye, and said, "I love you."

My parting words were, "Simon you don't have to be in pain. Call me when you get home if your pain is not under control."

A few weeks later, on a Saturday morning, Roger and I were reading the newspaper, still in our robes. The phone rang, and it was Sue. She said, "Judy, Simon is in terrible pain. I don't know what to do. The doctor hasn't been able to help him." She was crying, and I could hear Simon in the background moaning.

I asked if they would mind if we came to see them, and they gratefully accepted the offer. On the long drive to their home, I felt sick at the thought that the same old poor-pain-control saga was torturing my friend. Even though it was a bright clear day, the drive seemed to last forever.

When we arrived, we found both of them in a state of exhaustion and misery. They had been awake all night trying to make Simon comfortable. Sue and I went into the kitchen and sat down at the table, where she proceeded to put her head down and cry. After she was able to calm down, she showed me the medications Simon was on. As so often happens, they were not only incorrect dosages but also incorrect medications for the type of pain Simon was having.

Next, I went in to see Simon. He was sitting on the couch with his head in his hands. His spidery legs extended from his gray cotton bathrobe, and as he lifted his head, I saw the puffy eyelids and the strained expression on his face. I could hear the despair in his voice as he said, "If I had the strength I would walk down to the lake, go in, and not come out. I can't live like this, in all this pain. I even thought of getting in contact with Dr. Kevorkian."

The room filled up with silence as Sue let out a small gasp in response. I knew by the set of his lips and the look in his eyes that he meant what he said.

As I walked toward him, he started to cry. I gave him a hug and took his hand and sat down on the chair across from him. I asked him some questions about his pain and asked if he would mind if I called his physician. He said that it would be all right with him then added that his physician was on the board of directors at the nearby hospice and that he should know all of the needed information about good pain management. I assured Simon that his pain should and could be managed and that I would put my best effort into the project. He began to cry again, but this time it was with relief; he knew that he could get through all of this if he wasn't in such pain.

I called Simon's physician, who agreed with my suggestions and called the prescriptions in to the local pharmacy. Roger and I stayed with Simon while Sue went to pick up the medication. Interestingly enough, it wasn't a narcotic that Simon needed but a specific medication for the severe nerve pain that he was having. He started feeling some relief within two hours after taking it.

Before we left that afternoon, I asked Simon some goal-related questions. "When your pain is under control, *and it will be,* what do you wish for?" He stated that their first grandchild was due in a few months and he wanted so badly to be here for that. He also added that he would love to get together with all of his tennis friends one more time.

I promised him that when he was ready I would get everyone together; all he had to do was call me and tell me when. They both were smiling when Roger and I left that day. Knowing that Simon's suffering was about to stop, they now had some hope to hold onto.

I had had no problem getting his physician to agree to proper pain analgesia for Simon. Now, you ask, *Why didn't his physician know what Simon needed?* Good question. If a physician with a connection to hospice couldn't manage his pain, how in the world can we expect other physicians to know good pain management? I was just grateful that this physician's ego wasn't so large that he wouldn't take my suggestions. I have often called physicians who blew up over the phone because I had the audacity to suggest to them what their patients needed.

Two days later, Sue called to say that Simon was pain free! What a thrill it was to hear the good news. Our friend was still dying from his cancer, but his life had been returned to him.

The following week Simon called enthusiastically to say he was ready for his party. I made a few calls to some of the other wives, and one week later Simon and Sue arrived at the tennis club to find eighty of their tennis friends waiting to greet them—some they hadn't seen in years. Simon was overjoyed. What a party! He and his friends talked about old times, and told "Simon" stories and jokes. One of the guys wrote a poem for Simon and read it to all of us. A group of us sang a song that one of them had written about our friend Simon. Simon was the happiest guy there that night. He was still dying of cancer, but he was able to live life to the fullest now that his pain was gone.

Simon's little granddaughter was born a few weeks later—another of his goals reached.

As he neared the end, Simon had more setbacks, but his spirit remained intact and alive. He also had some good times. The local hospice had provided the added care he needed for his family to keep him at home, which was where he wanted to be. I was fortunate to have spent a few more days in his home helping with his care just before he died. We miss you, Simon!

Balancing the Benefit vs. the Burden

The wise man lives as long as he should, not as long as he can. We will think of life in terms of quality, not quantity. Life, if thou knowest how to use it, is long enough.

Seneca
Epistulae Morales, AD 60

The secret is in knowing when to say enough is enough. I do believe in miracles, but they will only occur if the spirit is strong and has some fight left in it. When survival depends on medical interventions that are not affecting a cure, are a burden for the patient, and many times just pure torture, why do we keep trying to hold onto the body while in the process destroying the person inside? Just because we can do one more treatment, try one more procedure, or insert another tube doesn't mean that we should. For whom is this being done? In many cases, it's for the family or the physician, not the patient. Whose life is it anyway?

Death takes only a moment. You breathe out and you don't breathe in—that is death. On the other hand, dying can take a very long time. Should we expect that time to have some meaning in our lives, or are we well served spending that time hooked up to tubes in a sterile environment, frightened and miserable? If we are able to address this issue as the benefit versus the burden, then our treatment options can become our friend rather than our enemy.

It is often very difficult to know when to stop treating the disease that a person has and begin to treat the person who has the disease. These differing approaches can sometimes go hand in hand, but far too often that isn't the case. Even with the best of care, there comes a time when the treatment becomes more of a burden than a benefit for the patient. That decision is best made by the patients if they are able to voice their needs.

They should receive support for their decision, not opposition, because only they know how much of a burden the treatment is for them. If another round of chemotherapy will give them a few more months of life, will those months be filled with excessive hardships brought on by the treatment? If so, would they prefer to spend the rest of their lives (however long that will be) doing what they want to do and where they want to do it rather than spending that time debilitated by the treatment?

Often, the treatment at this stage can be worse than the disease itself. For the patient, then, extending life becomes more of a burden than a benefit. The same can be said for patients who can no longer speak for themselves. That is why advance directives are so important.

The reality of dying can stop us, teach us, heal us, and perhaps even change us. If debilitating treatments are continued right up until the very end, we can lose the opportunity and the energy to discover and do what really matters. When physical healing isn't possible, one of the things that really matters is the healing of relationships while the dying still have the time and energy to do it. This can make a tremendous difference in the lives of those left behind as well as help the dying person to find some peace before the end. I have been privileged to witness this healing in families on more than one occasion, but never have I felt it more profoundly than in my own family.

Dad

Those who think that the disease must be cured in order for healing to take place don't understand that there is more than one type of healing that can occur when a person is ill. The healing that took place between my dad and me before he died had a significant, lasting impact on my life and, I believe, helped him to die more peacefully.

My dad and I had never been very close. I hardly ever lived up to his expectations, which were strongly related to money and power. I reminded him too much of my mother, whom he left for another woman after thirty-eight years of marriage. He left Mom with very little money and even less self-esteem. I was disappointed in him, and our contact was limited after the divorce. I finally decided that my mother needed me much more than my father did, and I tried to stand by her side through the bitterness and depression that followed their breakup. She moved close to my brother for a few years and then lived near me for the remaining years of her life. My dad and I remained separated—not only emotionally but also by the 1,100 miles between our homes.

Three years after my mother's death, I received a call from my father's neighbor. My dad (age eighty-four) had been in failing health for a year since his second wife had died. I had tried to visit him several months before, but he had not wanted to see me. My sister, who lived even farther away from Dad than I did, had remained in close contact with him and was aware of his health status, or so she thought. As it turned out, neither of us knew how poor his health had really become. We both thought that he was generally okay since he was still living alone in his house and was able to get out for his activities. He even had a girlfriend.

Dad had fallen the day his neighbor found him on the floor. He was bleeding from open wounds on both legs but refused to go to the hospital. He told his neighbor to call his daughter, the nurse, and she would know what to do. The neighbor promised to stay with him until I could get there. I was fortunate to find a flight that same day, and within three and a half hours, I was in his home. It was snowing when I left Ohio. When I got out of the taxi at my dad's house, the warm Florida sunshine, however, was the only welcome I received.

My dad greeted me with a frown on his face and wanted to know what took me so long to get there! He looked thin and pasty, and his gray hair was tousled. His legs were wrapped in towels, and the chair he sat in dwarfed his slight body. The bleeding had stopped, but he was in terrible condition. He was dirty, and the house smelled of urine.

My dad, a professional, had always been a proud man, and though he hated to admit it, he needed help. My first priority was to get him some medical attention. He again refused to go to the hospital, but I was able to get him to see a doctor, who gave me orders for medications and home-care services.

For three days I did the best that I could to stabilize him. I bathed him, dressed his leg ulcers, did what I could for the huge ulcer I discovered on his tailbone, and gave him his medicine. I transferred him in and out of his wheelchair, a task he said I would never be able to do. "This is what I do all the time as a nurse," I told him over and over again as he questioned my abilities.

The hardest part in all of this was trying to figure out the right thing to do for my dad. During this time, my sister had come in from California. There was a lot of discussion regarding Dad's condition and what to do about it, but in the end it was up to me to come up with a workable plan. I spent hours putting together an arrangement for home care supplemented by visits from friends and neighbors to provide the care Dad would need.

By the third day, however, I had seen enough of Dad's true medical condition to know that he could not stay in his home by himself even with home-care support. By this time, my brother and his wife had arrived from their home a few hours away. Dad did not want to stay with them, and sending him to California with my sister was not an option. It was suggested that I move in and take care of him, but I had a job and a husband back in Ohio. Finally, Dad decided that if I couldn't move in with him, he would go home with me and see if my doctor could help him.

Those three days were very difficult, but the healing of our relationship had begun. I made arrangements to fly us both back to Cleveland, and we went to the airport that evening. I wheeled him on board the airplane and got him transferred to his seat and buckled in. He ordered each of us a glass of wine, and we both smiled as he held up his glass and waited for me to raise mine. As we clinked our glasses, he said, "To you, my wonderful daughter. I thank you and love you. I never knew you were so smart."

I was stunned but very pleased. My dad was eighty-four years old, and I could never ever remember him having said "I love you" to me.

My husband met us at the airport, and we took my dad straight to the hospital, where my physician met us and examined him. Dad spent the next month in the hospital—twice undergoing surgery for the severe ulcers that had developed earlier. When the surgical treatment had run its course, he was sent to a nursing home for rehabilitation.

Dad was very ill and was not getting any better. The severe infection that he had developed at his home continued to get worse in spite of an intensive antibiotic regimen. His quality of life had deteriorated so much during that time that at this point he was just existing without truly living. I watched as the fluids were pumped through tubes into him. As a result, his lungs became so congested that he could hardly breathe. His body became swollen from the excess liquids, magnifying his discomfort. It was difficult to stand by silently as this torture continued.

Modern technology was not serving my dad with compassion or dignity. Even though it continued to prolong his life, it was prolonging his pain and suffering. The benefit from the "care" he was receiving was negative. The burden from this same care was excessive. It served no one well, especially my dad. It was becoming more than I could take.

My brother and his son, a physician, both living out of the state, had not visited Dad at all during the time he was with me. Even so, they both insisted that all available invasive and curative medical interventions be continued. So often we see this in families. We call it "the kid from California" syndrome. This is the son or daughter from out of state (or just out of town) who hasn't been home for a while and is feeling guilty and insists that "everything be done" whether it is warranted or not. They usually get their way because by now the patients can no longer speak for themselves, and the medical profession is afraid of a lawsuit.

As my dad's physical health failed, so did his mental health. Soon after he entered the hospital, we spent a lot of time talking about his wishes and what he would want if he should become unable to speak for himself. I was glad that we had these conversations because now I knew what he wanted and what sort of existence was acceptable to him. I could then make decisions based on his values and beliefs. As his spokesperson, I finally said, "Enough is enough." By then my sister had arrived from out of town, and she agreed with me.

We brought him home on hospice, played his favorite Dixieland music, and kept him comfortable and clean until he died. By the time I brought him home, his response was very limited, but there was still a lot to be done to care for his spirit. The music we played was his favorite. He was touched and cared for tenderly by those who loved him.

The total time from my going to Dad's home until he died in my home was three months. He was very ill that entire time. It was, however, the best time for my dad and me and our relationship. A healing occurred for both of us. We loved each other like never before. He told me that he was sorry for how he had treated me and that he was proud of me. Many times he told me that he loved me and thanked me for taking such good care of him while he was ill.

Some people die with the same bitterness they have carried with them all of their lives. Others can heal and obtain peace in the process. This lesson illustrates that dying can change us and teach us what really matters. What a gift those three months were for me! It healed all of the hurt that I had carried into my adult life. For a few years after Dad died, my brother refused to speak to me. He had wanted everything possible done to keep our dad alive, but I knew that it wasn't what was best for Dad. It is sad when families split apart during a death in the family. I missed my only brother, but I don't regret for a minute what I did for my dad. It took a while, but my brother and I have mended our relationship.

One patient I nursed on our hospice program hadn't seen his daughter in nineteen years. Her step-mother called her when he was put on hospice, and she came home and helped to take care of him until he died. They also healed their relationship as many others have. Dying time was a gift for all of them, as it was for me. It's satisfying to know that healing a relationship can erase all the anger and pain that we may carry with us. I only think of my dad now with love. Death and healing—an oxymoron? I don't think so.

LESSON 9

Futile "Care"

Only in the United States of America has death become an option.

Dr. Joann Lynn
Americans for Better Care of the Dying

Futile care isn't care at all. It is best described as medical treatment that not only does not accomplish its desired effect but in the process causes more harm than good. Over and over again, I wonder why such treatments are continued even when advance directives are in place to stop this foolishness.

For terminally ill persons and their loved ones, dying should never have to be a brutal experience. When it is said, "Everything humanly possible was done to keep the person alive," often, much has been done to destroy the spirit. In a medical environment where prolonging life through the avoidance of death is more highly valued than the reduction of suffering, it can be very difficult to maintain control over how we die. When the quality of life is poor and survival unlikely, the coercion to continue aggressive attempts to cure the disease or to keep the body alive must give way to what the *patient* wants.

Even when patients have made out their living wills, those directives are not always honored by some health care institutions and sometimes not even by family members. This is an appalling abuse of trust. Why can't a patient's wishes be carried out when those wishes have been clearly stated in writing, especially when his or her life is nothing more than physical existence and is filled with misery and suffering? If patients are unable to speak for themselves, it is imperative that they have strong-willed advocates who really know what they want and are willing to honor and will—as is sometimes necessary—fight for their wishes.

Most life-prolonging treatments, futile as they may be, are reimbursable within our health care system. This makes a lot of money for physicians, hospitals, and nursing homes. For too long I have seen nursing home patients receiving speech therapy, physical therapy, and other treatments that add nothing to their quality of life. Yet they are dying alone, in pain, and with crushed spirits. The spirits of their loved ones are crushed too. I call this futile care, and the cost to our nation in suffering and wasted health care dollars is simply ludicrous.

Rick

It was just before lunch when Rick called the office. The secretary said, "Judy, there is a man on the phone who has some questions about hospice. He isn't sure if we can help but wants some information." I picked up the phone.

Rick was distraught. He explained that his seventy-four-year-old mother, Carol, had been alone since her husband died eight years ago. She had been living in her own home and managing quite well until four months ago when she suffered a major stroke. She had been in a nursing home ever since. Now it was no longer the stroke, but her medical care, that was the problem. "My father was placed on life support for several months before he died," Rick told me. "My mother was certain that she did not wish to have that experience, nor did she want me to go through it again."

Two months after her husband's death, when she was still in good health, Carol had gone to her local hospital and picked up an advance directive for health care form. This form is available to anyone, free of charge. It is a legal document that defines our wishes for end-of-life care if we should ever become unable to speak for ourselves. Carol had completed this form, naming Rick as her spokesperson.

Carol had been working in her garden when she suffered the stroke and had been steadily declining since then. She no longer recognized Rick, was paralyzed on her left side, and could no longer swallow her food. Rick said he had been called to the nursing home that morning for a meeting with his mother's physician, her social worker, and a nursing coordinator.

"I was told that since my mother was no longer able to swallow, it was the policy of the nursing home to send her to the hospital to have a feeding tube inserted. I told them that I couldn't allow that to happen. My mother has a living will (advance directive) stating that if she was not able to speak for herself, she did not want a feeding tube inserted in her."

Rick also told the three health care workers that Carol had appointed him on a legal document to be her spokesperson should she not be able to speak for herself on these issues. "The coordinator said that if my mother remained in their facility, I didn't have a choice—it's their policy."

Not only that, but the physician had looked at Rick with scorn on his face and replied, "What are you trying to do, kill your mother?" Rick had staggered out of that meeting not knowing what to do. As a last, desperate resort, he had called hospice.

"I really don't know much about this thing called hospice," he said, "but I figured that if you can't help me, you could maybe suggest some other program that can."

I sighed. Rick's story was like so many others. Only the names change while the faces and voices remain anxious, helpless, and distraught. I invited Rick to come to our office and sit down with me to see if we could come up with a plan to help him and his mother. Within twenty minutes he was sitting across the desk from me.

Rick was a handsome, athletic-looking man about fifty years old with flecks of gray in his hair. He introduced himself and immediately handed me his mother's living will and the other paperwork noting him as her spokesperson. He was trembling as he said, "Judy, I'm not trying to kill my mother. I'm just trying to follow her wishes. She doesn't know anyone now. She just lies there and stares and moans. I hate to see her like this. It's been four months, and she's not getting any better. What can I do?"

I smiled kindly and said, "Rick, it was wrong for the doctor to say that you are trying to kill your mother. He had no business saying that. You and I both know that you are just trying to honor your mother's wishes. If he won't allow you to refuse the feeding tube, you have a right to fire him and find another physician who will." Then I told Rick that he also had the option of transferring his mother to another nursing home. He looked at me with stunned disbelief.

"I didn't think that I could do that," he said.

"You most certainly can," I replied.

Here was a middle-aged, smart, college-educated man who didn't understand that he had the power to do what he believed was right. I just shook my head and silently chastised the medical profession and the American way of dying. I see this over and over. Americans just aren't aware of their rights. Usually, such conversations take place in nursing homes with elderly spouses who feel even less empowered than Rick did. I wonder, sadly, how many family members agree to the agony and indignity of the feeding tube simply because they don't know that they have another choice.

When Rick asked me if I would help him find new arrangements, I picked up the phone and made several calls. Within two hours, an ambulance was picking Carol up from one nursing home and taking her to another. The physician I had called had done this for other hospice families with the same problem. That afternoon, this new physician met with Rick after her office hours. She became Carol's physician in the new nursing home, ordered hospice comfort care, and affirmed Rick's decision.

Carol lived for eleven days in comfort, with her only child, Rick, at her bedside. Standing behind him were the support and care of hospice and an understanding and compassionate physician. Carol's wishes were honored, and so were Rick's. He felt so supported that he came into the hospice office a week after his mother died and has been a volunteer for hospice ever since.

I can only imagine the gripping agony of his grief and anger if he had not called us. What a terrible legacy that first physician would have left with him.

Rose

After delivering a hospice presentation at a large retirement community gathering, I was approached by one of the social workers from the facility. "Judy," she said, "there is a couple that would like to speak with you about hospice before you leave. Her mother is a resident in our nursing home. They heard you speak tonight and stopped me to ask if you might have the time to talk with them." I replied that I would be happy to. With that, she handed me the chart of the resident in question.

I sat down and perused the chart as I waited for them. I quickly found out that the resident's name was Rose. She was eighty-six years old, and she had been in the facility for the past five years. Her main diagnosis was advanced Alzheimer's disease. She no longer walked or talked and for the past two years hadn't recognized her family or any of the staff at the facility.

In a matter of minutes, I looked up to find a middle-aged, well-dressed man and woman approaching me. I remembered seeing them in the audience as I did my presentation just a short time before. I also remembered that he looked very intense as he listened to me. They introduced themselves as John and Amy and sat down at the table with me.

John began the conversation by stating that he was very worried about his wife, Amy. As she sat next to him in silence, he told me about his wife coming to the facility seven days a week to feed her mother. Each meal took her one and a half hours to complete. Even with this special care, her mother's health was declining. He felt that it was time for his wife to come to the realization that her mother was dying. He also shared with me that his wife's health was failing and that he was afraid he would lose her before her mother died.

I turned to Amy, who looked at me with tears in her eyes. She told me that she couldn't just let her mother starve to death and that it took that long to feed her. I asked her if she thought her mother would want to live this way. I asked her if she and her mother had ever talked about her end-of-life care. She said that when first diagnosed with Alzheimer's, her mother had told her she didn't want to live when she could no longer function and take care of herself. I asked Amy if she thought her mother would be satisfied with the way her life was now.

"Goodness, no!" she exclaimed.

Then I asked her, "Amy, what is the worst part of this for you?"

She replied, "Coming here three times every day and knowing that it isn't making my mother any better."

I continued, "Do you think you are doing these feedings for your mother or for yourself?" She replied that she was probably doing it for herself but that she didn't know what else to do.

I asked her how she would feel if her children sacrificed their health and marriages to do for her as she was doing for her mother, who, by the way, continued on her way to death curled up in a fetal position, unable to speak or recognize any of her family. Her mother had been to the hospital by ambulance four times in the last six months—twice with pneumonia and twice with a urinary tract infection. Each of these times, her mother had been totally frightened and agitated by the change in her location and the haste of the ambulance ride. All four times Amy had stayed with her mother while she was in the hospital.

Her husband looked at her and confirmed his fears. "I am so afraid that our family is going to lose you. Your nerves are just about shot. We haven't been able to enjoy our retirement or our grandchildren. Please, listen to Judy before it's too late. Your mother's life is over. She doesn't even know when you are here. Why keep prolonging the inevitable?"

Her reply was, "I don't know."

John continued, "She wouldn't want to live this way. Why do you insist on keeping this up?"

She looked at me with tears in her eyes and stated that she didn't know what else to do. Could I help them?

I took her hand in mine, looked into her tear-filled eyes, and said, "Amy, this awful disease has won. Your mother needs very little now, but what she needs, she needs very badly. She needs for this to be over. She needs to be maintained as comfortably as possible. She needs for you, her daughter, to let go and let her die peacefully."

I explained that hospice could work with the facility to keep her mother comfortable at all times. Her mother could stay in the room that she currently occupied. Hospice would make regular visits to the facility to supervise and assist in her care. The next time her mother developed an infection, hospice would see to it that she stayed at the facility and received only comfort care. She and I both agreed that we wouldn't want our children to spend so much of their lives feeding us when food wasn't going to make us better. For the most part, it would just unnecessarily prolong the inevitable.

Amy actually looked relieved. "I just never knew what else to do. No, my mother would hate to live like this. Her dignity is gone, and she was always such a proud woman. She wouldn't want me to come here every day to make her eat."

She signed the papers for hospice care that night. She still came to the facility once a day just to be with her mother. Rose lived for fourteen days. She died quietly in her bed, with her daughter and family by her side. I can't help but think that Rose was happy to be relieved of this life she was forced to "live."

Pneumonia used to be called the old person's best friend. Now, because we can successfully treat the pneumonia with antibiotics, we can extend life, but not necessarily for good reasons.

LESSON 10

How to Remain Fully Alive with a Life-Limiting Illness

Choose this day to not simply be alive but to live.

Anonymous

The pain of the spirit can be just as disabling as physical pain. When the spirit is in pain, it is the person, not the body, who suffers. To your spirit, it is not as important when you will die as it is how you will live until you die. The spirit *must* be kept alive and well if you are to have any chance of making good use of your remaining time. Much can be done to make this happen if we understand what the dying person needs.

What do we really need at the end of life when there is no cure for the disease? My patients have taught me that this is what they need to keep their spirits alive while they are dying:

- To have value placed on who I am as a person
- Dignity
- Physical comfort (to be free of excessive pain and other disabling symptoms)
- Honesty, respect, and compassion from others
- Spiritual and emotional support
- To heal deep and old emotional wounds
- To remain as independent as possible for as long as possible
- To achieve my goals (what I would like to do or need to do before I die)
- To remain hopeful in some areas of the process
- Personal control whenever possible
- The caring presence of others
- The loving truth of others
- To have my loved ones supported as they take care of me

Mr. and Mrs. West

The first time I met Mr. and Mrs. West, they were both worn out, worn down, and ready to give up. He was dying of end-stage heart disease, and she was living with a broken heart. They had been married for more than fifty years, had raised four children, and were spending in misery what they thought would be their golden years together.

They lived in an area that once was in the country but was quickly becoming urbanized. New development was occurring all around them, but the trees on their property still blocked out the construction. The large windows throughout their magnificent, century-old home surrounded them with a marvelous view of their wooded lot. The house was filled with remarkable antiques, and the whole place had a unique charm about it. It didn't take me long to realize that the charm came from Mrs. West. The love in that home was everywhere. So was the sorrow.

The year before our hospice team made its first visit, Mr. West had been in the hospital more than he had been in his own home. He had given up the struggle to live and was at home preparing to die. He had told his physician, "No more hospitalizations!" I'm not exaggerating when I say that when I first saw him, I was pretty certain he would not live for more than a few weeks. He was very frail and weak and had all but given up his will to live.

Mr. West was a nice-looking gentleman who was more worried about his wife than he was about himself. He was soft spoken and sported a thin mustache that looked almost too perfect, as if it had been drawn on with an eyebrow pencil. He spent most of his time in bed.

Mrs. West, on the other hand, was strong and in control. She was a petite, spirited woman with sharp, angular features. Her hair was mostly gray, and she wore it in a knot on top of her head. Most of the time, when she was not taking care of her husband, she was in the kitchen baking or cooking. That was her way of handling the stress. The house usually smelled of cookies baking or yeast rising.

Mr. West had frequent episodes of chest pain, difficulty in breathing, and severe coughing. Mrs. West took very good care of him but lived in fear that the next attack would be his last. Their children lived nearby but were busy with their own families and work. They helped whenever they could, but most of the time the Wests were alone.

The first few months he was on our hospice program, Mr. West's heart condition declined slightly, but his spirit began to heal. Once he and his wife found out that he would not have to go back to the hospital and that we would help both of them through the difficult times, his will to live returned. This also did a great deal to help his body do better.

Our hospice team made numerous trips to their home each week—daytime, evening time, and in the middle of the night as well. We helped them through the bad times when symptoms were severe. We helped them through the fears and anxieties that occur with so many of the families we serve. We had family meetings with their children and spouses and with the grandchildren as well. Each time Mr. West's chest pain worsened, we went to the home to assess the situation and then contacted his physician, who would adjust the medication to control the pain. We taught his loving wife how to care for him as newer, sometimes technical, equipment was needed. Just knowing that hospice would pay for all of these new medications and equipment helped to decrease their anxiety. They knew that we were but a phone call away.

As their fears diminished, their hope returned, and Mr. West's spirit took on new life. After he had been on our program for six months, we found that he would stabilize for a while and then would have another episode of severe pain or develop another debilitating symptom that required our immediate attention. Most of his symptoms were related to chest pain and difficulty in breathing, but at one point the skin on his legs broke open, and we had to take care of that.

Medicare regulations say that hospice patients are supposed to die within six months, but Mr. West was having none of that nonsense. When his one-year anniversary with hospice arrived, he invited the entire hospice team to a restaurant for lunch to celebrate with him and his wife the fact that not only was he still alive, but most importantly to them, one year and no trips to the hospital. He ordered wine for all twenty of us who were there that day. As he raised his glass, he toasted, "Thank you all for giving my wife and me another year of love."

Mr. West got out of the house a lot during that first year on hospice. His wife or children would take him for drives in the park or out to lunch. He even danced at his son's wedding! Most of the time he had to use a walker, but he was a happy man. Those outings were followed by days of being too weak and tired to get out of bed, but he said it was worth it. Because of the hospice care and support he received, his spirit had recovered and had become strong. He was able to remain fully alive even though he still had a life-limiting illness.

The beginning of his second year on hospice was more difficult for both of them. We knew that Medicare would not be happy with us for keeping him on hospice, but we just couldn't find the heart to discharge him from our program. Within a few months into that second year, Mr. West died. Three weeks before his death, he used what little energy he had left to go to his granddaughter's birthday party.

Many family memories were created during that fifteen-month period—lasting memories for a wonderful family and for our hospice team. I am convinced that when you help someone *feel* better, it often allows that person to *do* better. Mr. West was a prime example of what a difference good end-of-life care can make in the life of a family. You see, hospice doesn't necessarily mean that death is soon—it means that there is no cure for the disease and that the time remaining is limited.

Shortly after Mr. West died, our fears were realized when we got a letter from Medicare stating that we would be required to pay back the money they had paid for his hospice care. We checked with our hospital records and found out that for the year before he became a hospice patient, Medicare and his private insurance had paid the hospital $300,000 for his hospital bills. For the entire time that he had been on our program, it had cost Medicare less than $7,500! It had cost Mr. and Mrs. West nothing. We had paid for all of our services and all of his medications and equipment out of the money that Medicare had paid us for his care.

We took Medicare to court and won. Mrs. West had insisted upon testifying in support of our case. She stood up in court and said, "It's not my husband's fault that he did so well on hospice, it's not my fault, and it surely is not hospice's fault. Please pay these people what is owed them, as I could have never done it without them." We still keep in contact with Mrs. West. She is now a part of our hospice extended family. She even bakes cookies for us.

In my estimation, every good hospice program should have a patient now and then who is discharged from the program for a cause other than death. By helping people feel better, they often do better. Perhaps renewing their spirits strengthens their immune systems. Whatever causes it, occasionally a temporary reversal can occur—call it a "miracle recovery" of sorts that allows patients to be discharged from hospice and returned to a more normal life for some period of time. As encouraging as this may seem, their terminal condition has not disappeared but has only been fortuitously postponed. When the disease once again asserts itself, hospice will be waiting to help the patient through the final journey.

Tom

Tom was a thirty-year-old divorced man whom I first met while he was being treated for advanced cancer in the hospital where I worked. He had already been there for ten days the morning we first met. I found him curled up on his bed in severe pain. His chief complaint was that he was in terrible pain and no one in the hospital seemed to know what to do about it. Tom rated his pain as a ten on a scale of zero to ten. He was just miserable.

Occasionally, a physician or nurse would call in hospice to help manage a patient's advanced cancer pain. I explained to Tom that hospice was very knowledgeable about pain management and that was the reason for my visit. While we talked, I found out that the pain was controlling his life. He said that he would be satisfied if his pain was reduced to a tolerable level, but he wanted to remain as alert as possible. I shared that we might not be able to completely eliminate his pain but that it was always possible to make it much more bearable. Within two days, Tom's pain was not gone but was well managed to his satisfaction.

I visited him those first two days, and we talked a lot during that time. I found him to be an intelligent, handsome young man with a magical spirit. He was personable and had a friendly smile that welcomed me warmly whenever I entered his hospital room.

I enjoyed those visits. Since I was about the age his deceased mother would have been and he was about the age of my two sons, we found much to talk about. His mother had died when he was a young boy. He and his sister and their father had then moved in with their grandparents. His grandparents were both dead now, but he and his sister had remained very close. Tom had been married for two years and divorced for one, but he and his ex-wife, Mary Ann, remained friends. They had a darling three-year-old daughter named Brianna, who lived with her mother in another state. Tom had numerous pictures of his daughter in his room at the hospital.

Tom had not worked for the past year. He had been too sick with the chemotherapy that he was taking. He was well informed about the disease he had. He knew the tumors were growing rapidly and that there was no cure available. He said, "I'm just tired of fighting it."

Now Tom had to decide whether to keep up the treatments that his physician recommended. These treatments might give him another month or two of life but would also produce the side effects that he found to be so awful. Or he could go to his sister's home and try to make use of whatever time he had left.

His sister's priest had been visiting Tom in the hospital and was encouraging him to continue his treatments. By focusing on the disease, those around him had totally lost sight of Tom and his needs. Tom was confused as to what God would want him to do. Together, we explored the possibility that maybe some of his pain revolved around issues of loss and emotional suffering. He agreed that this was a very real possibility. I suggested that he might need his remaining time and energy to deal with these issues. Also, I suggested that the best place to do this "work" might be away from the hospital, someplace where life was not centered on cure and treatment.

It was clear to me and soon became clear to Tom that the focus of his goals was not the same as the professionals who were caring for him in the hospital or the priest who was visiting him on a regular basis. He decided that he would rather go to his sister's home, where he could live the life he had left on his own terms. With the help of hospice, he went home from the hospital the next day.

Maintaining control of his remaining time was important to Tom, and he actually did quite well at home for a month and a half. He was very happy throughout that time. The more control he gained, the stronger he became and the better he felt. His dying time was truly a personal experience. He gained a sense of meaning and purpose during that time. The hospice chaplain visited him regularly and journeyed with him on his quest for spiritual health and peace. I felt that this was a small miracle in itself. He was so young.

His main concern was Brianna. He loved his daughter very much and had been active in her care before he became so ill. Hoping for a cure when his cancer became more aggressive, he had moved away from his daughter to his sister's home near a large medical center and from there had ended up in a hospital bed.

One day while I was sitting with Tom at his sister's, I asked him the question I often ask my hospice patients: "Tom, what is the worst part of this for you?"

He answered without the slightest pause, "My daughter is so young. There is so much that I want to say to her. Will she remember me? Will she ever know how much I love her? Will she ever know what joy she brought to me?"

Mary Ann had brought Brianna in for a visit the week before, but he was left with the knowledge that this little child was still only three years old and that he might not ever see her again. I knew in my heart that even though we had been successful in taking away his physical pain, much of his spiritual pain remained.

I replied, "Tom, no one is gone until they are forgotten. Why don't you make a video to tell your daughter all of the things you want her to know? Then she will never forget you."

He responded, "Judy, I don't have any money to get a camera." I asked him if he would like me to work on that, and he replied that he would be very grateful if we could manage to find some way to do it.

One of our volunteers was only too happy to help Tom with his project. For the next three weeks, Tom became very involved with his video to his daughter.

As we helped him to feel better, he also did better. He was able to transcend this most difficult time in his life in order to share his love with his daughter. His sister often said that she knew this was what kept him going. This became his goal, and it served him well. He finished his last gift to his child just before he lost his battle with cancer.

I can only imagine what a gift this was to his daughter and what it will mean to her as she grows up without her father's presence. I know that it brought Tom much joy just being able to do it. Medication alone was not the catalyst that brought Tom to some peace before he died. There were also the human connections and communications and a revived spirit that gave him life while he was dying.

LESSON 11

How to Nurture a Dying Spirit

When we honestly ask ourselves which persons in our lives mean the most to us, we often find it is those who, instead of giving advice, solutions, or cures, have chosen to share our pain and touch our wounds with a gentle and tender hand. The friend who can be silent with us in a moment of despair or confusion, who can stay with us in an hour of grief and bereavement, who can tolerate not-knowing, not-curing, not-healing, and face with us the reality of our powerlessness, that is the friend who cares.

Out of Solitude
Henri J.M. Nouwen

The dying have taught me so much. If I could speak for them, this is what I think they would want me to say to you.

Even though I am facing death, I am still living. Don't look at me with pity.

I may need to talk about my thoughts and fears in order to cope with them. Just listen and accept me without trying to change or fix my mood. You don't have to have answers for all of my difficulties.

Respect and accept me as a whole person, not as a disease. (I have had persons say to me that they need others to know that they are still the same person inside even though they look so different from when they were well.)

One of my deepest fears is that I will be reduced to the helplessness of an infant. Help me to take care of my own needs as long as I can—even little things. (It is compassionate to help others do what they cannot do for themselves. It is not compassionate to take over the life or death of the patient or the caregiver. When we do for others that which they can do for themselves, we risk depriving them of their dignity and self-worth. Compassion is more about empathy than sympathy or pity.)

Always remember that I'm still living—I'm not dead until I'm dead! (Hearing is the last sense to go.)

If I can respond, speak directly to me. Look at me, not at the floor or the walls or at someone else in the room.

Tell me ways that my life has touched yours. (We all need to know that our lives have made a difference to someone. This adds value to our lives, is good medicine for our spirits, and gives us a sense of accomplishment.)

Help my family to share their memories with me. Bring out photographs, do a life review, help me to remember and share with me the stories that reflect the time that only you and I had together.

Don't be afraid or ashamed of tears—yours or mine. I need to grieve this loss that I feel.

If you don't know what to say, that is okay. You really don't have to say anything, but if you do, let it be sincere. (Sometimes, a human touch, a hug, or a kiss means more than words.)

Be honest. If you are not honest, I will imagine the worst, and my anxiety level will increase.

Give me as much control over this entire journey as you can. I am losing control of every aspect of my life, so don't take away the things that I can still do for myself.

Even though you may not agree with my decisions, unless there is a reason to think that they are unsafe, please respect and honor them.

If I am in denial, that is okay. Denial is my way of protecting my spirit at this point. Just give me some time to come to grips with reality. I know the truth, but I'm just not ready or able yet to face it. Let me decide how to manage this heartache that I feel.

Let me be with whatever comforts me. Sometimes that may mean being in my own bed, in my own home with my animals and familiar objects around me. (Being in a hospital's sterile environment and being forced to follow the hospital routine is not supportive to a dying person. I have often gone into a home only to see the dog on the bed, the bed by the window with birds at the feeder, and flowers in bloom that the dying person had planted before becoming so ill.)

Be reliable. Please don't abandon me.

Help my family and loved ones to understand that I am doing my best. If I don't eat, that is okay. Eating is not going to change what is happening to me. If my energy level is decreasing, it is because of the disease that I have. Let me use my energy for what I want to do. If I want to spend time with a friend instead of doing exercises or going to the hospital for an X-ray, let me do it. It will nourish my spirit, which is really all that is important at this time in my life.

I don't want to simply give up and die, but when I am tired and sore and want to stop fighting whatever it is that is destroying my body, let me go and wish me well. I need this not only from my family but also from my physician, my social worker, my nurse, my clergy, and others who are important to me.

What can you say to a dying person? This is always difficult, but I have found some things that you might say to help make it easier. There are also some things you should not say. Some of these suggestions also apply to the caregiver.

"I don't know what to say—what has the doctor told you?"

"I don't know how you feel. Help me to understand what this is like for you."

Never say, "I know how you feel," or, "Everything happens for a reason; it is just a part of God's plan," or, "Don't talk that way," or anything close to, "I feel your pain"—because you don't. Don't compare another person's experience with the patient's situation.

Very often, it is how persons feel when they are with you rather than what you say to them that gives them comfort. The entire visit doesn't need to be centered on the person's illness. Even too much sunshine can burn. But avoiding the issue of the person's illness is not the answer either. To pretend that all is well is not supportive of the patient.

"What is the worst part of this for you?" (Handle the response with care—to downplay or sugarcoat it is unfair. We all deal with loss differently. This may be the only chance the person has to express his or her greatest fears and deepest worries or thoughts.)

"Do you want to talk now?" (Don't interrupt or give advice early in the conversation; it stops dialogue. Offer advice only if asked for it.)

"Would you like for me to sit with you or to go?" (Sometimes just sitting with them is the best medicine. Sitting brings you closer to their eye level, which is the best place to be. If there is no conversation, don't try to fill up the silence with stories or activities in your life. It is okay to just sit and be with the patient.)

If you are having a difficult time, don't change or avoid the subject. Just say, "I'm having a hard time talking about this right now. Can we talk about it later?"

When you are with people who are dealing with life-limiting illnesses and you are struggling for the right words to say, ask them if they would like to share with you something about their life stories. This can promote spiritual wellness in them that they didn't know they had. Telling personal stories at the end of life can be a profound spirit-healing experience. When others take the time to listen to these stories, a personal connection is created. This helps the dying to deal with the grief they are feeling in losing their lives, the illness they are living with as they die, and the other challenges they are facing.

Unfortunately, because it is often a time-consuming process, our health care system places limited value on the importance of just being with patients and attending to their spirits. Because of staff shortages and financial bottom lines, the medical profession and those who pay them concern themselves mostly with medications, radiation, chemotherapy, X-rays, MRIs, and any other treatment that directly supports their attempts to cure the disease. Yet as we take the time to connect with the sick and dying, we nurture the wellness of their spirits and possibly improve our own at the same time.

When done well, end-of-life care will affirm a dying person's life and our own as well. What else could be more important if the body cannot be cured? Our greatest gift then becomes our willingness to be in the presence of the dying person, empathetically as well as physically. While we are with them, we can listen and enter into the unknown with them. This goes beyond the words we speak to them. It has more to do with *being with* them rather than *doing for* them. I call this process "presencing." At first, it may be uncomfortable for us, but as we become more confident in ourselves and in the health of our own spirits, we will find it is not as difficult.

Presencing can never be forced on other persons, but if they sense in us a willingness to engage, it will be invited. It becomes an open door for the dying to show their vulnerability. It gives them comfort to know that someone has chosen to be with them in their suffering and dying. The sharing of their burdens not only reduces their suffering but can be a tremendous help to their spirits. Presencing is the act of one human spirit embracing another human spirit. It may not require a lot of time, but it does ask that we stay in the moment regardless of how uncomfortable it may be.

ONE FINAL NOTE

Heroes

Joy-filled presence, there are many days when the last thing I want to do is smile or have a good laugh. This caring for a dying one is tough. It takes its toll on the human spirit. Help me to find moments in the day when I can smile. Help my loved one and me to laugh together, to find the little joys in life that sustain and uplift us. Remind us often that you are with us.

Joyce Rupp

Caregivers

The caregivers of the world are my heroes. To visualize a hero, most of us think of people who have had much said about them and have received trophies and awards. Some of us think of movie stars, sports figures, and politicians.

I have witnessed the twenty-four-hour-a-day heart-wrenching love and devotion provided by care-givers. This has taught me that being a true hero is usually a silent and lonely affair. It is unaccompanied by the media glory of acknowledgment. There is no award or trophy and sometimes not even a thank you. Sometimes these heroes don't even have the time to care for themselves. Simple things, even brushing their teeth, take a backseat to the immediate needs of the loved one. Most of the time their hearts are hurting as they attempt to do things for their loved one that they never in their wildest imagination dreamed they would ever have to do for anyone. Yet they just keep doing it.

Many of them are elderly and frail themselves and have no experience in nursing. They ask for little and do so much. They go on despite fear, worry, anxiety, and lack of sleep. They choose to do their hero work without the thought of how it is affecting them and even praying that it will never end. Each of their stories is different, yet each of them touches my heart and strengthens my belief that heroes are those who "just do it" and will receive their glory just by doing it.

Faith

When my good friend Faith, who was in her midfif-ties, married for the second time, her friends and family were delighted. Faith was and still is a beautiful woman. Chuck, her new husband, was a handsome man in his early sixties. They made such a wonderful couple. Both were educated, well spoken, fun loving, and very grateful for the life they had found together. Faith's adult children loved Chuck, if for no other reason than the fact that he dearly loved their mother. Her new husband was a man of character. He was devoted to her and her four children, grandchildren, and even her elderly mother. His first wife had died of cancer. He also had adult children of his own, and the two families blended well.

Faith and Chuck lived a wonderful life together for eight years. They lived on an island near Savannah, Georgia, where they enjoyed many of the same interests. They traveled, played golf, and started plans for a new home. Then, quite suddenly, Chuck became ill with a terminal lung condition. Both families were devastated. Faith had found such joy with him in their new life together, and now it would all too soon be gone.

I spoke with Faith many times during Chuck's illness. I tried to give her emotional support and information concerning his care. We did this by long distance because they lived hundreds of miles away from me. His illness progressed slowly over a period of six months, but each change in his condition brought a new crisis. During one of his frequent hospital stays, his physician told them that there was nothing more that could be done.

Faith was overwhelmed. Chuck wanted to be at home, but Faith wasn't sure she could take care of him, even though she had a nursing degree. I mentioned hospice to her when she called to give me this sad news. At first, she didn't want to even talk about hospice; to her it meant only death. But of course, to me it meant life—the opportunity to live life to the fullest within the limited time remaining. We talked a lot during that time about what was possible and how she could get the help she would need to keep Chuck at home.

Life wasn't easy (it usually isn't for caregivers). Faith told me how she would be up all night taking care of Chuck when he had a bad night. She told me how she had to attend to his personal needs, helping him into the bathroom, bathing, lifting, positioning him in bed, attending to his breathing treatments, and on and on. Her back had become very sore from all of the lifting she had to do to help Chuck. To make matters worse, with so much to do and so much on her mind, she was not sleeping well.

Finally she realized and admitted to herself that she couldn't do it alone anymore. She called hospice and was surprised and relieved to discover the amount of help they could give to Chuck and her. Hospice took over the role of bathing and most of the lifting.

Soon Faith was feeling better both emotionally and physically.

It is so frightening, both to the patient and to the caregiver, when the patient can't breathe. Hospice taught Faith how to care for her husband during those difficult times, and she was able to overcome her fear and help Chuck. They worked through those periods with the medications and treatments that Faith was now trained to give.

There were times when she called me just to cry or talk, and I listened. I thought the most difficult part of Chuck's illness was that they just couldn't believe this was happening to them. They loved each other so much and were now living their worst nightmare together. Through it all, they never gave up hope that somehow Chuck would get well. But this dream didn't come true, and Chuck died in his home with his wife holding him in her arms.

Shortly after Chuck died, I received a note from Faith. She told of the time before Chuck died and how she treasured that time with him. I will share a part of the note with you.

> *Chuck's daughter, Holleigh, was with me when Chuck died at seven p.m. Holleigh and I just cried so hard. We prayed and cried some more. We sat with Chuck until the hospice nurse came at nine p.m. I continued to sit with Chuck and rub his chest (his beautiful chest). I kept touching him. It seemed so natural for*

me. I was so glad that he was still with us. I really felt that he was. It was a very spiritual experience. Talking over him just felt so natural, also.

The hospice nurse wanted to clean him up, so we left the room. When she was finished, one of my neighbors came over with her rosary beads. She and I said the rosary over Chuck. It was wonderful. We both cried some more.

The funeral guys arrived about eleven p.m. They wanted to know if I wanted to see them take Chuck out of the house. I told them yes and don't cover his face. They were very compassionate. Before they put Chuck on the stretcher they let me say good-bye one more time while he was still in the bed. They closed the bedroom door, put him on the stretcher, and wheeled him out through the dining room and out the front door with me at his side. This all just seemed just so right. I still think that it was right. I still relive it a lot. They let me kiss Chuck one last time before they took him away.

I just wanted to share this with you, Judy, because it was such a sad and beautiful thing. Chuck and I had six months together here at home, and we shared a lot with each other. Thank God for that time. I cannot imagine what sudden death is like. It has to be terrible. We had our crying spells together, and he would say, "I am going to miss you so." With the help of hospice I knew what to expect, and it made it so much better.

I have made a list of things to be grateful for during Chuck's illness. I will share these with you *sometime. There are pages. God is good. As I read this I do not think that I made it sound as wonderful as it was. Just being with him those hours before they took him away meant so much to me.*

Faith's story is not unique. I have never in all my years of doing hospice had caregivers say that they were sorry they took care of their loved ones at home. Yes, it is hard. Yes, the nights sometimes seem endless. Yes, you do get very tired and even irritable. Yes, it's sometimes frightening and troubling. But that's just what heroes do!

Volunteers

Volunteers are some more of my heroes who are important to the hospice concept. They can do much to add to the quality of life of dying patients and their loved ones. They receive no pay for their tireless work, and they always come back for more.

Jim

Jim, one of our male volunteers, truly became an inspiration to me and to many of our families. He took patients fishing "one last time," even though Jim didn't like to fish. He took them to doctor visits, watched them for caregivers who needed a break, and always went that extra mile for the families he served. I'll always remember the day he called me at the office to tell me that "his" patient asked him to take him for a ride in the park to see the fall leaves. While they were on their ride, Jim's patient asked him if he could have one last beer, and off to the patient's favorite bar they went!

One of Jim's patients, Mr. G., was from India. Jim studied the man's culture so that he could better understand his needs. He learned that in India the dying want to be out of doors and on the ground as they are dying. Mr. G. was in a nursing home for the last several months of his life. Jim would visit him there, take the mattress off of his bed, and lay it on the floor, where they would sit back to back to hold Mr. G. up. Jim would take him out of the nursing home in a wheelchair for long periods of time until Mr. G. would say it was okay to go back in.

Even in the fall, when the weather was cool, Jim would wrap his patient in a blanket and outside they would go. The staff at the nursing home couldn't believe how much Jim honored Mr. G.'s beliefs. There was a mutual understanding between these two men. As was his wish, Mr. G. died peacefully on the mattress on the floor, with his family and Jim at his side.

I have seen Jim doing the laundry for the spouse who was at work while Jim stayed with the patient. He went to the store, did the dishes, picked up the house, and did anything else he saw that needed to be done.

He would do almost anything to help a family "as long as it isn't illegal or immoral." To me and to the many, many families Jim helped care for, he is a hero!

Conclusion

> Studies show that the course of 100 percent of medical/surgical patients regardless of treatment modality will *without exception* ultimately terminate in death.
>
> Dabney Ewen, M. D.

It has been said that death is the king of terror. Death, however, takes only a moment; you breathe out and you don't breathe in—that is death. On the other hand, dying can take a very long time, and depending on how you approach it, it can be either a miserable, sometimes terror-filled experience or an enlightening adventure.

The secret is to remember that even though the body is dying, the spirit can remain alive and well in the process. I believe that we have a moral responsibility to nurture the spirit of a dying person. When there is light in the spirit, there will be hope and strength in the person. If there is hope and strength in the person, there will be peace and hope in the home. This allows for the inevitable to occur with the least amount of anguish.

As we face the end of life, the spirit is always changing. Sometimes it is very difficult to keep it from getting weak. We must work together to help those who are suffering. We must help them to keep their spirits alive and well. We may be the only companions they have during this time, so it becomes our responsibility to be kind and compassionate and to add peace and dignity to the process. We need to bear witness to their lives and bear witness to their dying.

I have learned from my patients and their loved ones that when they are supported, honored, and well cared for, there are tremendous opportunities for growth at the end of life. It is possible to create wonderful memories for those who are left behind.

I have seen that, given a little time, with appropriate end-of-life care that relieves pain and provides comfort, spirits can make remarkable recoveries and patients are able to make productive use of the time they have left. To do this, they need to have control over some aspect of their lives. They need a place of peace where someone is not always pushing them to eat more or urging them to get well, all the while disregarding the fact that they are dying. Understanding *their* needs can help us make the process of dying more humane.

The truth is, if the body can be comforted physically and emotionally, the spirit will not be injured and in fact, may grow. Unfortunately, too many dying persons are never afforded this opportunity. Ninety-eight percent of people polled stated that they would rather be at home and comfortable at the end of their lives, and yet over 50 percent of those with a terminal illness still die in a hospital—often alone and in pain. This time would have been better spent caring for their spirits. In my estimation, when we lose sight of this, we have caused more harm than good.

We can see in the same institution the best and the worst of medicine. We see wonderful cures, but when the cures aren't achieved, unrelieved suffering is often the result. People assume that physicians are schooled in death and dying and end-of-life care, but in truth, little training is received. Much of the medical profession could benefit from education in these disciplines, but there is a natural reluctance among physicians to accept this.

We are not required to use all that is medically available just because we can. Sometimes it is more humane not to go for that last series of treatments. There are institutions, physicians, nurses, and family members who will admonish the patient not to give up on a treatment even though they wouldn't want it for themselves if faced with the same decision. I believe that prolonging life is not as important as alleviating suffering when there is no cure for the disease.

Dying, in and of itself, is not a medical problem that needs to be solved. It is how we die that needs our attention. Dying is our own personal experience. It is as unique as our DNA—no two are alike. Each of us will have our own personal needs and desires that can be fulfilled only if we make them known.

The essence of life is not found in the shells that are our bodies. The essence of life is in our spirits. Most importantly, remember that as we die, we are not human beings having a spiritual experience; we are spiritual beings having a human experience. The human body may succumb to disease or disability and lose its usefulness and become a burden long before its eventual death, but the human spirit can remain alive and well up until the very end.

listen|imagine|view|experience

AUDIO BOOK DOWNLOAD INCLUDED WITH THIS BOOK!

In your hands you hold a complete digital entertainment package. In addition to the paper version, you receive a free download of the audio version of this book. Simply use the code listed below when visiting our website. Once downloaded to your computer, you can listen to the book through your computer's speakers, burn it to an audio CD or save the file to your portable music device (such as Apple's popular iPod) and listen on the go!

How to get your free audio book digital download:

1. Visit www.tatepublishing.com and click on the e|LIVE logo on the home page.
2. Enter the following coupon code:
   23f5-950b-cb6e-a236-88d5-155f-bf81-e11d
3. Download the audio book from your e|LIVE digital locker and begin enjoying your new digital entertainment package today!